Hobart Paperback No. 23

CHALLENGE TO THE NHS

Challenge to the NHS

*A Study of Competition in American Health Care
and the Lessons for Britain*

David G. Green

Published by
THE INSTITUTE OF ECONOMIC AFFAIRS
1986

First published in September 1986

by

The Institute of Economic Affairs
2 Lord North Street,
Westminster, London SW1P 3LB

© The Institute of Economic Affairs 1986

ISSN 0309-1783

ISBN 0-255 36194-7

Printed in Great Britain by
GORON PRO-PRINT CO LTD,
CHURCHILL INDUSTRIAL ESTATE, LANCING, WEST SUSSEX
Set in 'Monotype' Bembo

Contents

Preface

by LORD HARRIS OF HIGH CROSS

The *Hobart Paperbacks* were devised as studies of medium length between Papers and books in which economists would analyse the relationship between theory and policy. In particular, authors were invited to consider the circumstances which encouraged or inhibited the translation of ideas into political action.

It was appropriate that this new IEA series was launched in 1971 by Professor W. H. Hutt with the title *Politically Impossible . . .?* in which he argued that economists should pursue their analysis to its logical conclusion and not dilute it to fit fallible preconceptions about whether their proposals were politically acceptable. Subsequent *Hobart Paperbacks* have applied this astringent approach to such contentious issues as British membership of the EEC, the role of trade unions, foreign aid, farm subsidies and, most recently, to the proposal for an educational voucher to replace direct state finance and provision of schools.

Hobart Paperback 22 is a characteristically forthright challenge to the defenders of the most politically sacred of all sacred cows. The National Health Service appeared, at least until recently, to be the most cherished example of successful collectivist enterprise, in defiance of the elementary precept that economic goods could not be efficiently supplied or consumed without a price being demanded and paid. (Except for its public-goods element, medical care is no exception.) Other IEA authors have persisted in questioning the NHS model throughout the quarter of a century since Professor Lees wrote an early Hobart Paper (No. 14), *Health through Choice*, in which he concluded:

'The fundamental weaknesses of the NHS are the dominance of political decisions, the absence of built-in forces making for improvement, and the removal of the test of the market'.

Professor Lees, plainly without much hope of being heeded, refrained from offering a blueprint but pointed towards far-reaching reforms that would 'diminish the role of political decision and enlarge

ix

the influence of consumer choice'. Thus governments should move away from taxation and free services to private insurance and fees. They should disperse the control of hospitals, cease to determine doctors' incomes, make a percentage charge for drugs (except for life-saving drugs and poor patients), and end control over entry to medical schools by financing students through loans rather than grants.

The next landmark was the *Occasional Paper* by my colleague Arthur Seldon published in July 1968 to mark the 20th anniversary of the NHS and prophetically entitled *After the NHS*. With luminous clarity, he demonstrated that if state finance were channelled to people with low incomes, government could avoid the escalating cost and declining satisfaction that must forever dog universal provision at zero price (then costing £1,600 million compared with £18,000 million in 1985). If the better-off majority were not trusted to insure privately from higher and rising post-tax incomes, he offered the model of compulsory third-party car insurance or an earmarked health voucher to ensure compliance.

With a prophetic vision that shames the complacency of myopic party men, Mr Seldon gave three reasons why the NHS must yield ground to competing private health care. First, as incomes rise expectations would continue to grow beyond the state's capacity to finance. Secondly, the contrast would intensify between 'privately-financed, market-provided abundance in everyday consumption and publicly-financed, state-enforced stringency in welfare services'. (If Mrs Thatcher had grasped that central truth, would she ever have said 'The NHS is safe in our hands'?) Thirdly, he foresaw that other countries would demonstrate the advantages of choice, competition and freedom from detailed governmental control, and that such deficiencies that remained in the market could be more easily remedied, not least by enforcing competition, rather than through the deformities of a monolithic nationalised, politicised, health service.

In this and subsequent Papers, Arthur Seldon has stubbornly emphasised and embroidered the earlier warning expressed succinctly by Dennis Lees in 1961:

'On the longer view, the most acute danger of the NHS is that it will prevent the emergence of more effective methods of medical care'.

The increasing scope for higher spending on health care (and other services) was revealed in three field surveys between 1963 and 1970 published first in *Choice in Welfare* (1963, 1965, 1970) and brought together with a fourth in a *Hobart Paperback* (No. 13) entitled *Over-ruled on Welfare* (1979). Asked if they would accept a voucher for two-thirds of the cost of health insurance (£60 in 1978) and add one-third from their pocket, a clear majority (57 per cent) of a national sample of 2,000 heads of household said they would accept it in place of the NHS.

Dr David Green's study is a worthy addition to a distinguished line of other IEA publications. Instead of elaborating the earlier analytical critiques of the NHS, Dr Green devotes most of his space to reporting on research into the remarkable recent developments of the lively health-care market in the United States. Fortified by wide reading of documents and academic interpretations and by three recent strenuous visits to the USA, he is able to present an absorbing, variegated picture of recent changes in the organisation and finance of the services pro-vided by entrepreneurial doctors, hospitals and insurance organisations.

Perhaps the major reason that ears have been so long closed to radical reform of the failing NHS was the spread of travellers' tales about the shocking neglect of sick, low-income Americans who lacked insurance cover as the only passport to hospital. Dr Green explains that, although such stories are generally untrue, they are not without a grain of verisimilitude. Thus, any serious casualty can be assured of emergency treatment, but uninsured patients must expect to be moved to a state hospital when their condition has been stabil-ised. The author does not regard this arrangement as satisfactory and acknowledges a necessary but neglected role for government to bring all American citizens within financial reach of the medical care that is generally rapidly outpricing what is available in Britain.

The author's wide-ranging and well-documented report also lends some credence to popular impressions of American doctors performing unnecessary operations and their patients (or corporate insurers) being brought towards bankruptcy by the inflated bills. But the interest for economists and other serious students, though not for superficial writers and party hacks, is in the reasons Dr Green explains for such abuses. The chief explanation can be summed up in the word 'mon-opoly' which, as an earlier Chicago economist once warned, 'has no use, save abuse'. Thus our author painstakingly demonstrates that the principal failings of American medical care have not been the result of competitive markets but of the doctors' 'professional' closed shop which restricted entry of medical students, raised charges, resisted change and frustrated consumer choice.

Since most medical bills are met from private insurance provided for employees by their employers, the usual market corrective of reduced demand did not operate to discipline excessive costs. Once again the competitive market could not be blamed when customers are denied awareness of cost and rendered indifferent to over-charging by monopoly suppliers. In view of the well-advertised 'scandals' of American medicine, particular attention should be given to Dr Green's account of the break-up of the doctors' monopoly and the way the corrective of competition has begun to discipline costs and in the process to check unnecessary medication, which will remain rampant throughout the NHS so long as doctors, nurses, administrators, patients, politicians and hypochondriacs remain indifferent to the costs of alternative therapies.

The resulting American innovations could never have been predicted by the brightest economists, let alone by British politicians, doctors and medical bureaucrats forever lamenting the lack of resources to appease their price-less medical monster which must never be defiled by money. Only a free market, as Hayek's 'discovery procedure', could yield the wealth of experimentation which Dr Green outlines in Section VIII. Even the most ideological apologist for state monopoly must surely be impressed by the almost bewildering evidence of developments in the services provided by hospitals (both 'non-profit' and for-profit), insurers (likewise), and doctors, whether specialists or GPs, and given by medical auxiliaries when freed from the self-serving subservience to doctors. Under pressure to contain costs, Dr Green reports that employers and insurers increasingly require the patient to pay some part of the bill, just as British insurance companies reduce their premiums if motorists pay the first £50 or so of car repairs. Insurance companies are also refining methods of comparing the performance of doctors and the costs and effectiveness of alternative treatments. For their part, patients are increasingly offered a choice between 'health maintenance organisations', 'preferred provider arrangements', second opinions, one-day surgery centres, home care agencies, walk-in clinics and many more variants, including brand-named treatments!

Mothers are encouraged to return home backed up by a family aide one day after normal childbirth, at a quarter of the cost and often with less disruption or emotional disturbance than staying several days in hospital, which the NHS lavishly and needlessly indulges. And the author emphasises that the impact of competition on experimentation and innovation is far from spent.

To return to the theme of the *Hobart Paperbacks*, I judge one of Dr Green's most interesting disclosures to be the confirmation that some British economists specialising in health care have come to deprecate the analysis of competitive alternatives to the NHS as wasting time on 'politically impossible' solutions. Instead of examining how far and in what ways competition and pricing might remedy the worst deficiencies of the NHS, they swell the chorus of misplaced 'compassion' that health is 'different' and join in demands for more money whilst acknowledging they do not know whether the NHS could be judged efficient.

As an economist who has avoided the temptation to make forecasts, which have so often brought the prophet into disrepute, I am emboldened by Dr Green's illuminating study to predict that the NHS will never reach its 50th anniversary (in 1998) in anything like its present form. In the approach to the next election, the latest spasm of discontent may wring more resources from a hard-pressed Government. But without any means to secure either efficiency in supply or economy in demand, additional spending is more likely to inflate costs than to increase real output. There will be no lasting redress of grievances. Instead, governments will continue to be seen as restricting the growth of a major part of the service sector by discouraging increasingly prosperous families from spending their own money as they would wish.

Not the least evil of political control in health care has been the power conferred on governments to prevent 'informed' discussion of policy. A recent example was the appointment in 1976 of the Royal Commission into the NHS under the chairmanship of Sir Alec Merrison to which Arthur Seldon and I submitted evidence that was not even acknowledged. In a published conversation with Peter Hennessy, Dr David Owen, with characteristic candour, admitted that as Minister of Health he had rigged the Commission to ensure it

> 'was not going to come out with a powerful minority report [which] would oppose the basic principles of the National Health Service . . . I would claim it was done for higher motives. But it was rigged'.[1]

---

[1] *The Great and the Good*, Policy Studies Institute, London, 1986, p. 15 (reproduced from the transcript of a BBC Radio 3 broadcast, 'The Good and the Great', 4 February 1985).

The dispassionate observer is entitled to ask how strong is the case for such a major aspect of policy if its political master considers it needs to be protected from truly independent impartial assessment?

The constitution of the Institute requires its Trustees and Directors to disclaim any commitment to Dr Green's analysis and conclusions. However, my colleagues and I are sufficiently impressed to contemplate creating a special research unit to extend the study of alternative policies for improving medical care. Meanwhile, I have no hesitation in commending this outstanding *Hobart Paperback* to students, teachers, policy-makers and commentators as a major contribution to public discussion of the future of the NHS and the alternative arrangements that may supersede it sooner than now seems likely.

June 1986   RALPH HARRIS

Author's Foreword

Could Britain improve upon the National Health Service? Many of us think of the NHS as symbolising the essential decency of Britain, so anyone who asks whether a competitive market would be preferable to the NHS is in danger of being dismissed as 'uncaring'. I hope to show that, on the contrary, if the argument of this book is adopted, every person's chances of getting the best health care available, rich and poor alike, will be improved. Nor will the reader find any reluctance to assign to government the task of underwriting the material security of its people. In a civilised society the poor should be protected by government action. That is not at issue. What is, is that we are failing to take into account the contribution a competitive market might make to the supply of health services. I say this not out of some ideological attachment, but because, as I will show, the weight of evidence suggesting that competition improves the quality of service enjoyed by the consumer is overwhelming.

I did not reach this conclusion lightly. I spent the best part of 10 years in the Labour Party, over five as a Labour councillor, and at one time held a quite different view. But the evidence, both from our own recent past and from similar countries overseas, that we could improve on the NHS if we introduced greater competition is very persuasive. I present some of it here, so that the reader can judge whether it is really as convincing as I have come to believe.

This study is the fourth in a series which examines whether a competitive market in health would make an attractive alternative to the NHS. *Mutual Aid or Welfare State* (1984) looked at Australian health care before large-scale government interference began in the early 1950s, and *Working Class Patients and the Medical Establishment* (1985) examined primary health care in Britain before the NHS. *Which Doctor?* (1985) examined the legal and institutional structures that buttress professional power and stand in the path of competition in Britain today. It is now conceded by some defenders of the NHS that these studies of pre-war health markets in Australia and Britain show that health care was supplied through the market with fewer imperfections than had previously been supposed.

The response of some critics, however, has been to accept the validity of the new historical evidence, but to deny its relevance to today's health-care debate. Medical technology, they say, has so transformed medical care that historical evidence has no contemporary value. This reaction is an overstatement, but it is true that historical evidence alone is insufficient to support generalisations about the potential for a competitive market in Britain. I have therefore begun to look afresh at the contemporary scene in Britain and America. The natural first choice was America, where despite considerable distortions due to government interference (the government finances well over 40 per cent of health care), the market still plays a major role. My study of the American health-care market continues, but the evidence from that country appeared to be of sufficient importance to justify publishing this preliminary account for the non-specialist reader.

June 1986   DAVID G. GREEN

The Author

DAVID G. GREEN was born in Norfolk and educated at the University of Newcastle upon Tyne, 1970-73, where he studied Political Science and Sociology. He undertook postgraduate research at the same university, which awarded him a doctorate in 1980. Whilst a post-graduate he lectured part-time at Newcastle upon Tyne Polytechnic. From 1972 until 1981 he was a Labour Party activist, serving as a Labour councillor on Newcastle city council from 1975 to 1981. He held office as chairman or vice-chairman of a number of committees or sub-committees, and served as a governor of three schools. He is currently a Research Fellow at the IEA, having been a Research Fellow at the Australian National University, 1981-83.

Dr Green is the author of four books: *Power and Party in an English City* (London: Allen & Unwin, 1980); (with L. Cromwell) *Mutual Aid or Welfare State: Australia's Friendly Societies* (Sydney: Allen & Unwin, 1984); *Working Class Patients and the Medical Establishment: Self-Help in Britain From the Mid-Nineteenth Century to 1948* (London: Temple Smith, 1985); and *The New Right: the Counter-Revolution in Political, Social and Economic Thought* (Brighton: Wheatsheaf Books, forthcoming). The IEA has previously published his *The Welfare State: For Rich or for Poor?* (Occasional Paper 63, 1982), and *Which Doctor?* (Research Monograph 40, 1985). His work has also been published in journals such as *The Journal of Social Policy, Political Quarterly, Public Administration, Philosophy of the Social Sciences, Policy and Politics,* and *Economic Affairs.*

Acknowledgements

I owe a considerable debt to a number of American scholars and health officials who gave up their time to discuss American health care with me. I am especially grateful to Bob Helms of the Department of Health and Human Services for guiding me through the American health-care maze from the beginning, and my thanks are no less due to Rosemary Kern of the American Enterprise Institute for help well beyond the call of duty. Particular thanks are also due to Professor Clark Havighurst of Duke University Law School for a most stimulating discussion of antitrust law, and to John Goodman of the National Center for Policy Analysis in Dallas for giving so freely of his time.

My thanks are also due to Bill Goldbeck of the Washington Business Group on Health, Sam Mitchell of the Federation of American Hospitals, Wayne Bradley of the American Medical Association, Jack Meyer of the American Enterprise Institute, Peter Biggins of LTV in Dallas, C. A. 'Chuck' Fiedler of Rockwell and the Dallas Business Group on Health, Charlotte Crenson of the Blue Cross/Blue Shield Association, Paul Ginsberg of the Rand Corporation, Chip Kahn of Senator David Durenberger's staff, Cheryl Austein and Stuart Schmid of Health and Human Services, Elizabeth Gee and Barry Costilo of the Federal Trade Commission, Pamela Mittelstadt and Kathy Michaels of the American Nurses Association, Beth Fuchs of Senator John Heinz's office, Warren Greenberg of George Washington University, and Rebecca Kupper of AMI.

I also thank the staffs of the American Hospital Association's Washington office, the Group Health Association of America and the National Medical Library. Special thanks are due to the staff of the Heritage Foundation in Washington for providing a most friendly environment in which to work during my final field trip to Washington, for which I must thank Ed Feulner, Burt Pines and Stuart Butler. And thanks are no less due to Andrew Amstutz, who served ably as my research assistant for 10 weeks in early 1986.

Several colleagues commented on an early version of this study. I have benefited greatly from criticisms made by my colleagues at the IEA, John Wood, Arthur Seldon and Ralph Harris, and thanks are no less due to two outside referees, Hugh Elwell and Professor Alan Maynard. Special thanks go to Larry Goldberg of the University of Miami for his valuable comments, made during a busy teaching term in London. Needless to say, I am responsible for any remaining errors or omissions.

Finally, I am very grateful to the Wellcome Foundation and the Wincott Foundation for contributing towards the cost of the project.

D.G.G.

Introduction

Arguments in support of the NHS fall into two groups. The first is the traditional demand-side argument that the government has a responsibility to ensure that the poor do not go without health care. The second focusses on supply-side arguments, holding that the market is incapable of supplying health services. In particular it is said that professional monopoly power is a permanent feature of the provision of health-care and that consequently the state should act on the supply side as a countervailing power to protect the consumer. Recent developments in America offer some important lessons for both the demand- and supply-side standpoints.

The Supply-Side Case

The striking reality today is that even among those economists who believe the case for the market in general to be very strong, there are only a few in favour of the market supply of health care. British health economists, in particular, are virtually unanimous in their approach. They are, almost without exception, committed to the maintenance of the NHS structure of tax finance and delivery of a 'uniform' service in kind by a near-monopoly state system. They frequently advocate piecemeal reform of the National Health Service, but rarely, if ever, question the foundations of the NHS edifice. This is not merely because the NHS is already in place, and therefore the unavoidable starting point for any realistic reformer. It is primarily because orthodox health economists believe that the chief rival to the NHS, the competitive market model, has little or nothing to contribute. Some are utterly dismissive of the market concept. For instance, according to one of the leaders of the prevailing orthodoxy, Professor A. J. Culyer of the University of York,

> 'health-care markets are always and everywhere so imperfect that the marketeers' image of the market for health is a completely irrelevant description of an unattainable Utopia' [Culyer, 1982, p. 27].

The chief reason this view is taken is that health care as such is said to be uniquely different from all other goods and services. A long list

1

of the unique properties of health care has been drawn up over the years, but three are thought to be of decisive importance:

(1) The monopoly power of the medical profession.

(2) The consumer's lack of information – which means that real consumer choice is impossible.

(3) The uncertainty of demand for health care – which necessitates health insurance, a type of insurance which has typically led to an undesirable escalation of costs because of '*moral hazard*'.*[1]

Other properties are listed below, but I devote little further attention to them in order to focus on the generally-acknowledged strong points in the orthodox analysis of health markets. For instance:

● Life itself may be at stake. Medical intervention is sometimes irreversible and, if mistaken, may leave the patient disabled or dead. (This characteristic clearly marks out medical care from many goods and services, though by no means all. It applies to other products too. A faulty car repair may result in a fatal accident. An unsafe toy may kill a child. A shoddy roof repair may lead to a fatal accident, and poor electrical work may kill.)

● Harmful externalities requiring government regulation may arise, as for instance, when a person fails to be inoculated against contagious disease and consequently puts others at risk. (There are relatively few negative externalities, and they can be overcome by relatively mild government intervention.)

● The market may fail to supply some 'public goods'. Again, this largely concerns contagious disease. A wider concept, the 'caring externality', has been suggested by Professor Culyer.[2]

The three main 'market failures' – professional power, consumer ignorance, and moral hazard – are said to be discoverable in both market and state systems of health care, because they are inherent in

---

*Glossary, p. 114.

[1] 'Moral hazard' is the name given to changes of attitude on the part of both doctor and patient which occur because the patient is insured. Once they have paid their premiums, patients may take the view that they want to 'get their money's worth' and consume more health care than they otherwise would; and the doctor, knowing that a large company is paying, may advise unnecessary treatment and/or inflate his bills.

[2] A discussion of this notion can be found in Sugden [1983]; also Culyer's reply in Culyer and Posnett [1985], and Sugden's rejoinder [1985].

the service itself. From that observation, orthodox British health economists infer that changing the public/private mix will make no difference [McLachlan and Maynard, 1982, p. 554]. They conclude that British scholars should therefore concentrate on resolving these 'failures' within the NHS and simultaneously desist from advocating market solutions. Implicit in this view is the belief that competitive markets are incapable of overcoming the special difficulties of supplying health care. Some economists go even further and accuse advocates of competition of wasting the time of their colleagues by continuing to advance a discredited argument [Culyer, 1982, p. 53].

NHS as a 'countervailing force to medical monopoly'?

Of the three main 'market failures', professional monopoly power is seen as an inescapably permanent feature of health care, and from this assumption it is inferred that the state must protect the consumer by direct control of the supply of health services. Professor Culyer, for example, argues that the NHS has the potential to control overmighty medical professionals. It could, he says, monitor their performance in the light of 'socially, not merely medically, determined objectives' [1976, p. 147]. Nick Bosanquet, his colleague at York, holds a similar view. Above all, he says, the NHS has been 'a countervailing force to the medical monopoly'. Originally, he believes, 'the most important part of this role was in reducing monopoly power over price' [Bosanquet, 1984, p. 49].

This *Hobart Paperback* questions the supply-side view. In Part 1 it looks afresh at the reasons for the doctors' monopoly in America, the chief source of unfavourable evidence about health-care markets. Is professional monopoly power the result of the inherent tendency of the market to monopoly, or is there a counter-explanation? Part 1 will also examine the extent to which the consumer's lack of information has been manipulated by the medical profession. Orthodox theorists claim that the doctors' monopoly is in part a consequence of the consumer's lack of information, but I will suggest that in reality it is the other way round: the consumer's lack of information is a result of professional power. The medical profession has controlled comparative information to render consumer choice ineffective; and it has limited the development of alternative forms of health-care delivery in order to restrict choice.

Similarly, Part 1 will examine the root cause of the third market failure, moral hazard. Again, orthodox theorists have neglected to examine in detail why the health insurance industry failed to control costs, preferring to assume that third-party health insurance in itself raises costs. But there is considerable evidence that, in the early days of health insurance in America, the industry did act in a cost-conscious manner, until it succumbed to a hostile campaign mounted by organised medicine that led insurers to abandon their efforts to contain costs.

The United States has usually provided the evidence for the conclusion that health-care markets do not work. And in America for a period until the late 1970s the producer was indeed in charge. Medical costs were escalating through the roof and unnecessary surgery was said to be commonplace. Yet now, in the mid-1980s, there exists a state of affairs which appears closely to resemble a competitive market. Large hospital corporations no longer charge whatever they please, but rather worry about retaining market share. Doctors are being forced to cut fees. New providers have emerged to compete with both hospital inpatient care and with outpatient departments. New insurance schemes abound. Part 2 describes these dramatic developments and explains what brought them about.

The Demand-Side Case

The main purpose of this *Hobart Paperback* is to survey recent developments in America and to explore their implications for supply-side theory. But, in addition to re-appraising the supply-side standpoint, I also briefly examine American experience in providing for the poor and elderly. I devote relatively less attention to the problems faced by the poor because I regard their circumstances as raising a largely moral question which is not in dispute in Britain. The government should in present circumstances prevent low-income families from being denied essential health care due to their lack of resources. In Britain we have already accepted this principle and it is not necessary, therefore, to repeat the arguments for protecting the poor as of right. The practical problem we face is how to introduce more competition for the benefit of all.

The American situation is a little different. The arrangements made by American governments for the poor and elderly during the last 20 years have been unsuccessful. The open-ended subsidisation of

Medicare (for the elderly) and Medicaid (for the poor) promoted sky-rocketting costs. Recently, the federal government has succeeded in putting a lid on rising costs, but a permanent solution has yet to be found. Moreover, provision for the uninsured poor through tax-financed county hospitals is discriminatory when set alongside the arrangements made to subsidise employer groups through tax concessions. In addition to being unfair, these subsidies are also imprudent. They give most to the well-off, and nothing to groups who are in most need, like the unemployed, and people who work for small employers without health plans; and their open-ended character encourages cost escalation. These issues are the subject of Section IX.

PART 1

The Rise of Monopoly in the USA

I. Restricting Entry

Using evidence from the 1970s, many British health economists have noted that professional monopoly power appeared to be a characteristic of all advanced nations. Professor A. J. Culyer, for example, observed that

> 'a strongly organised professional monopoly that controls entry to the profession, terms of service, permitted forms of advertising, disciplinary procedure, etc., is a *universal* characteristic of all developed countries (wherever they lie on the liberal-collective spectrum)' [Culyer, 1982, p. 37; italics in original].

Two main explanations for professional power are usually given. The first, according to Professor Alan Maynard, is that it is the 'natural inclination' of a competitive market 'to become monopolistic' [1982, p. 495]. The second reason is that the consumer is too ill-informed to be able to exercise real power of choice, and is thus driven into the arms of the producer. There are, says Professor Brian Abel-Smith, 'few fields of consumer expenditure where the consumer is as ill-equipped to exercise his theoretical sovereignty as in health services' [1976, p. 48]. Professor Culyer goes further. The marketeer, he says, 'betrays a naïve faith in the capacity of individuals to resolve their own problems'. The marketeer's image of a 'prototypical consumer shopping around for the best quality care at the least price, and getting it, is not a phenomenon that is anywhere actually going to be observed' [1982, pp. 38-9].

The 'market vulnerability' theory favoured by Professors Maynard and Culyer may be contrasted with the theory of 'state capture'. This questions whether professional monopoly is inherent in the market, and suggests instead that it is a result of government interference. According to Professor D. S. Lees, for instance, monopoly gains are 'potentially largest where a profession has achieved legal or effective monopoly through the political process' [1966, p. 46]. On this argument, professional power is a result, not of 'market failure', but of 'government failure'.

Today we have more evidence to test the two competing theories; not only historical evidence from both Australia and Britain [Green and Cromwell, 1984; Green, 1985b], but also strong new evidence from America.

The American Medical Association's Approach to Monopoly

The chief instrument of professional monopoly has been the American Medical Association (AMA). It was established in 1847, and by the turn of the century had already acquired its legendary power. In the early 1960s around 75 per cent of all US doctors were in the AMA, and, more significantly, about 90 per cent of doctors in private practice were members [Rayack, 1967, p. 2]. It was not until the 1970s that cracks began to appear. In 1971, for the first time in 50 years, AMA membership fell to around 50 per cent of doctors and has subsequently continued to hover around that level [Starr, 1982, pp. 398, 427]. From 1975 the AMA also faced mounting pressure from the Federal Trade Commission (FTC) to refrain from impeding competition. These interventions weakened the anti-competitive impact of the AMA, which is the subject of Section VII. First, I will describe how the AMA conducted itself up to the mid-1970s.

The AMA has long had a federal structure. At the base there are about 2,000 county medical societies. Until 1982, when direct membership was permitted, a doctor did not usually join the AMA direct, but rather the county medical society. The county societies in turn form part of the autonomous medical society in each state, which in their turn are the constituent associations of the AMA. Constitutionally, the 300-strong House of Delegates is the AMA's policy-making body, but it meets only twice a year and in reality the 15-member Board of Trustees wields effective power.

Dissent among AMA members has generally been suppressed – space in their journal has been denied to critics [Hyde et al., 1954, p. 946] – but the key to the AMA's control over members has been the power of the county medical society. Because its control reaches into the locality, the county society can enforce the AMA's *Principles of Medical Ethics*, often without the necessity to take formal action. Social ostracism can be decisive to a doctor, whose business depends crucially on being able to refer patients to specialist colleagues and on receiving such referrals. This power became all the more awesome as specialisation expanded. In 1940, 24 per cent of doctors described themselves as specialists. By 1955 the proportion was 44 per cent, and, by 1966,

69 per cent [Starr, 1982, pp. 358-9]. A doctor judged 'unethical' could also be made to suffer loss of advancement in hospital appointments or in his career generally. When such informal sanctions failed each county medical society had a 'board of censors' to enforce formal discipline. Members can appeal, with the AMA's Judicial Council having the final say, but it is bound by local findings of fact [Hyde *et al.*, 1954, pp. 949-50]. Consequently, most doctors have toed the line. As the authors of the *Yale Law Journal's* pioneering study of the AMA concluded, for the large majority of doctors defiance of the AMA meant 'professional suicide' [Hyde *et al.*, 1954, p. 953].

Local medical societies have also denied price-cutting doctors access to the Blue Shield medical plans described in Section IV. Similarly, local malpractice insurance companies have been used against colleagues who engaged in competition. In a country where doctors face a high risk of being sued by dissatisfied patients, the denial of malpractice insurance cover makes practice more expensive and, in the extreme, impossible. Commercial rates for non-county medical society members have often been 20-100 per cent higher, and some commercial companies have refused to give non-society members any cover at all [Hyde *et al.*, p. 951].

Controlling the Supply of Medical Practitioners

From the outset the AMA sought to monopolise medical practice, and its first objective was to establish a system of licensing. It lobbied in every state for the establishment of boards of medical examiners to administer examinations and to issue licences. By the turn of the century most states had succumbed and established a medical examining board which usually followed a policy identical to the AMA's. It became common for the state medical society to recommend or nominate appointees to the examining boards, and in one case the State Medical Society Board of Censors was the State Board of Medical Examiners [Hyde *et al.*, 1954, p. 959].

In the early years of this century, once licensing was firmly under professional control, the AMA gradually switched its efforts to controlling the accreditation of medical schools, thus enabling it more sharply to limit the number of doctors. In 1904 the AMA's Council on Medical Education was founded, and in 1906 it surveyed all medical schools and judged that 32 out of the total of 160 were unacceptable. In order to give their findings enhanced public credence, the AMA persuaded the prestigious Carnegie Foundation to repeat the survey. The outcome was the Flexner report of 1910 which recommended the closure of a number of medical schools. According to the report, only medical schools adjudged by the AMA to be class 'A' should be allowed to function. (Until 1928, the AMA classified medical schools as A, B, or C. After 1928 it simply listed those that were approved.) The result was that medical examining boards in most states, either by rule or habit, adopted the policy that only graduates of medical schools approved by the AMA or the American Association of Medical Colleges (AAMC) would be accepted as qualified for licensure. (The lists of the AMA and the AAMC were virtually identical.) The results were dramatic. In 1906 there were 162 medical schools; the number was reduced to 85 in 1920, to 76 in 1930, and to 69 by 1944 [Kessel, 1958, pp. 25-9].

This reduction was a mixed blessing. Some medical schools had turned out graduates with virtually worthless certificates. The disappearance of 'degree mills' was no real loss, but the cost came later. By pushing out the degree factories, medical school accreditation fell under the sway of the AMA, which soon turned this power to self-interested use. Rayack's authoritative study [1967, p. 70] concluded that the initial reduction in the number of medical schools was justified by the low standards prevailing in some, and that the sharp fall in the number of doctors was an unintended side-effect. But, during the depression years and subsequently, the AMA pursued a clear policy of deliberately restricting numbers to increase doctors' take-home pay.

In 1933 the AMA Council on Medical Education declared that America had a surplus of 25,000 doctors and called upon the AAMC to bring about a 'substantial reduction' in medical school enrolments to eliminate the 'overcrowding'.[1] The Council's secretary criticised the practice of enrolling students 'without any regard to the needs of the profession or the country as a whole' [Hyde *et al.*, 1954, p. 972; Rayack, pp. 73-76]. The AMA's appeal was not ignored. In each of the five years before 1934 there had been an increase in enrolments; for each of the six years after 1934 enrolments fell [Starr, 1982, p. 272].

Until 1942, the AMA and the AAMC had each accredited medical schools, but from that year they jointly established the Liaison Com-

---

[1] *JAMA*, Vol. 100, 1933, p. 1,425.

mittee on Medical Education to authorise programmes of under-graduate medical training. Henceforward there was a single monopolistic accrediting agency. During the war years the AMA relaxed its efforts to restrict numbers, only to fight vigorously the efforts of post-war federal administrations to subsidise medical training. In 1949 and 1950 the AMA reported the highest expenditure among all the groups registered under federal lobbying law [Hyde *et al.*, pp. 955-6]. It was opposed, however, by the medical schools, represented by the AAMC. From 1951, under pressure, the AMA reluctantly accepted federal grants for construction work where there was a 'demonstrated emergency', though it remained totally opposed to federal aid towards running costs. From 1958 the AMA finally conceded that there was a shortage of physicians, and accepted increased federal aid for construction work, but still opposed subsidies towards medical school running costs.

The AMA was then forced still further onto the defensive. Between 1958 and 1960 three official reports claimed that doctors were in short supply. The AAMC continued to favour federal aid, and, finally, in 1963 the Health Professions Educational Assistance Act was passed, under which federal building grants as well as loans to students could be made. The AMA continued to oppose federal support for the operating costs of medical schools until 1967, but by then pressure for federal subsidies had become irresistible. From the late 1960s federal monies flowed into medical schools on a huge scale (Section VI) [Campion, 1984, pp. 242-3].

The AMA claimed throughout that its opposition to federal subsidy was based on its hostility, as a matter of principle, to state interference. The expanding state, it said, was a threat to individual freedom. That its real aim was to diminish competition is revealed by its enthusiastic acceptance of federal aid for medical research after the Second World War. By 1958, with the AMA's blessing, government grants comprised 64 per cent of total medical school research expenditure. The reason, Rayack concluded, was that research subsidies increase the *demand* for medical services, whereas training subsidies increase *supply* [1967, p. 99]. Nor did the AMA oppose the Hill-Burton Act of 1946, under which hospital construction and renovation was subsidised. Indeed, it enthusiastically supported it because doctors benefited financially from improved hospital facilities.

Foreign Medical Graduates

One effect of the AMA's control of the supply of doctors emerging from US medical schools was a huge influx of foreign medical graduates (FMGs). From time to time efforts have been made to restrict immigration. During the 1930s there was an increase in the number of foreign doctors coming to America as refugees from European fascism, and additional restrictions were introduced in some states, with 22 admitting no foreign doctors at all.

During the post-war years the number of FMGs obtaining licences in the US was not very tightly controlled because American doctors were content to allow some immigrants to practise in order to fill unpopular vacancies, especially in mental institutions. But newcomers were excluded from lucrative specialisms by the requirement imposed by several specialty boards that candidates must be US citizens, which excluded immigrants for at least the five-year citizenship qualification period.

The sharp rise in medical incomes which occurred in the 1950s led to a search for cheaper substitutes, and foreign-trained doctors began to enter the US in large numbers. In 1950, 5·1 per cent of doctors licensed in the US were trained overseas (other than in Canada). In 1959 the figure was 19·7 per cent, rising to a peak of 44·5 per cent in 1973, and thereafter declining to 23·6 per cent in 1978 and 16·6 per cent in 1981 [BHPr, 1984, Table B-1-2]. But since the early 1970s about one-fifth of active physicians have been FMGs.

Foreign medical graduates are not only from overseas. The shortage of places in US medical schools drove increasing numbers of Americans abroad to train in the expectation of practising in the US on their return. In 1955, 2,056 US citizens sought medical education overseas. Numbers accelerated during the 1960s, and in 1978 the figure was 11,500 [HRA, 1982].

As the number of foreign medical graduates grew, the eligibility criteria for licences were tightened. In 1976 a more demanding medical examination, the Visa Qualifying Examination, was introduced to slow down the influx of foreign-trained doctors, and from 1984 a new two-day examination was introduced by the Educational Commission for Foreign Medical Graduates (ECFMG) and the National Board of Medical Examiners (established in 1915) to replace the previous qualifying examinations [BHPr, 1984, A-1-22]. The failure rate of FMGs has always been high. In the 1930s between 30 and 50 per cent failed licensure examinations. In the 1940s the failure rate usually exceeded 50 per cent, and in the 1950s it ranged from 32 to 55 per cent [CME, 1964, p. 168]. This was due to the poor training provided in some foreign medical schools, and not simply to the AMA's preference for restriction of the supply. A considerable number of US citizens who train overseas never qualify in the US. One study which followed up the careers of 550 Americans 10 years after graduation in a foreign medical school found that about 25 per cent never qualified [cited in BHPr, 1984, A-1-23].

Summary

From 1910 the AMA was able to keep a tight grip on the number of doctors being trained and hence to limit the supply of doctors in active practice. Because of America's traditional support for the free movement of citizens, the AMA found it difficult to control the influx of foreign-trained doctors, but its power to limit doctors' numbers was not seriously threatened until the federal government deliberately set out to encourage the training of more doctors from the late 1960s.

Specialists – Limiting Numbers and Supporting Monopolies

Doctors not only sought to control the total number of colleagues in active practice; they also tried to limit access to lucrative specialisms. The practice of voluntary certification of specialists dates from 1917 when the American Board of Ophthalmology was founded. By 1961 there were 18 specialty examining boards [ABMS, 1980] and in 1983 there were 23, which between them issued certificates of qualification in 57 areas of general or specialist practice. In 1980 about 50 per cent of all physicians in the US were certified by at least one of the 23 boards [BHPr, 1984, A-1-23].

The American Board of Medical Specialties (ABMS), a federation of the 23 boards, oversees the certification programmes. Its policy of discouraging overlap between specialisms tends to create a number of discrete monopolies. New specialist schemes find it impossible to get established without ABMS approval, thus giving established practitioners the chance to impede the emergence of alternative forms of health care [Havighurst, 1983, p. 308].

From time to time demarcation disputes occur. In the 1960s there was heightened conflict between GPs and specialists over the confinement of hospital privileges to board-certified specialists. Dr Letourneau, president of the American College of Legal Medicine, has given examples. Asked by the journal *Medical Economics* whether staff privileges were ever withdrawn from GPs *en masse*, he replied:

'Yes, typically this happens when a horde of surgical specialists moves into an area only to discover there's not enough surgery around. I've seen it affect four or five hospitals in the same community. Board-certified men tried to freeze out the competition completely, although local GPs have been there for thirty years doing good work'.

Similar conflicts occurred between specialists. Dr Letourneau said that 'Wherever specialties overlap, there's likely to be contention. General surgeons clash with gynaecologists. Plastic surgeons clash with nose and throat men'. He recalled a particular case

'where we decided to give all the fractures to the orthopods [orthopaedic surgeons]. No go. The general surgeons decided they just weren't going to hand over all those cases. Eventually there may be enough orthopods to change the ground rules and make them stick. Meanwhile, both factions have access to the disputed area of fractures' [Rayack, 1967, pp. 224-5].

The specialty boards lay down standards of training and establish minimum training periods which range from three to seven years. Eligibility criteria have also been used to restrict competition. For instance, Kessel found that membership of the county medical society was required before specialty board examinations could be taken. Many young doctors who, because they are just starting out, are likely to engage in price competition to attract customers, also want to obtain specialty qualifications, for this is a principal method of enhancing income. But to cut prices was to risk denial of county medical society membership which, in turn, closed the path to specialist qualification [Kessel, 1958, p. 32].

The chief claim to legitimacy made by specialty boards is that they improve and safeguard standards. But, as Rayack says of demarcation disputes, 'Clearly, the physician's income was at issue and not the quality of medical care' [Rayack, 1967, p. 225]. Some boards have also imposed citizenship requirements which have no direct link with competence; others have reserved the right to reject candidates for *any* reason, with no obligation to state the reason and no appeal allowed [Rayack, p. 221].

A number of studies have examined whether specialty board qualifications serve as a guarantee of quality. Rayack, for instance, found
this not to be so. Certainly he found it no safeguard against unnecessary
surgery, citing a study conducted by the Columbia University School
of Public Health and Administrative Medicine in 1962. A medical
audit of 406 hospital admissions was carried out: one-third general
surgery, one-third in obstetrics and gynaecology, and one-third medical. The report found that, of 60 cases in which a hysterectomy had
been performed, a review of the operative report and the pathology
findings indicated that one-third were operated on 'unnecessarily'
and that questions 'could be raised about the advisability of the
operation in another 10 per cent'. Of 13 primary Caesarean sections,
'the surveyor raised serious questions about the necessity for surgery
in seven'. Three-fifths of the 406 admissions received good or excellent
medical care, one-fifth of the cases were judged fair, and one-fifth
were felt to have received poor care. Patients under the care of physicians certified by a specialty board, or under the care of house staff
in voluntary or municipal hospitals, were judged to have received
'the highest proportion of optimal care'. But this was true only when
care was given in hospitals affiliated to medical schools. The care given
by 'certified specialists in hospitals unaffiliated with medical schools
or having no approved training programmes was not superior to the
care given by physicians without such qualifications' [Rayack, 1967,
pp. 217-8].

In April 1976 the FTC's Bureau of Competition began to investigate
whether physician specialty societies functioned as anti-competitive
trade associations. It set out to discover whether their licensing procedures went beyond quality control, which it acknowledged could
assist the consumer. The American Society of Plastic and Reconstruc-
tive Surgeons attracted particular attention on the ground that the use
of board certification unfairly restrained non-certified physicians from
practising.[1] The American Board of Medical Specialties and some
societies altered their regulations so that they could not be accused of
unfairly denying certification to applicants, and the FTC took no
further formal action.

---

1 *New England Journal of Medicine*, 28 December 1978, pp. 1,464-6.

II. Suppressing Knowledge

Until 1982 an important part of the AMA's monopoly strategy was severely to restrict advertising by doctors. Having established a single standard of qualification by controlling medical school accreditation and physician licensure, it was important to maintain the pretence that doctors were essentially all alike. This could be achieved only by forbidding any doctor from drawing attention to the differences between his services and those of his colleagues. According to the Federal Trade Commission (FTC), the advertising ban successfully deprived consumers of information about prices and types of service which they needed to make a rational selection between physicians.

The FTC's first case against the AMA, in December 1975, concerned the unlawful restriction of advertising. The case was brought against the AMA, the Connecticut State Medical Society, and the New Haven County Medical Association. The AMA's *Principles of Medical Ethics* did not explicitly ban advertising, but Section V urged that a physician should not solicit patients. A number of interpretations of the 1957 *Principles* by the AMA's Judicial Council made it plain that in practice all advertising was banned. In one case the Judicial Council had found that 'solicitation as used in the Principles means the attempt to obtain patients or patronage by persuasion or influence' [Avellone and Moore, 1978, p. 479]. When the FTC case came to court, examples were cited of how the rule was interpreted in practice. A clinic in Santa Clara, California, was typical. It wanted to offer employers a scheme to prevent and treat industrial injuries, but found that each time it sought to make its service known to employers the county medical society told it that the AMA code of ethics prohibited physicians from sending out leaflets or brochures about their services or approaching local employers in any other way [FTC, 1981a, p. 90].

The control of advertising is closely related to the concealment of information in malpractice cases. For many years doctors cultivated the tradition that members of the profession do not criticise each other in the presence of outsiders, and especially patients. In addition to making it difficult for the patient to judge the relative merits of doctors, this professional solidarity has proved particularly harmful to patients when doctors have refused to testify against colleagues accused of negligence in malpractice cases. In the past, some doctors who gave evidence in court found that sanctions were applied against them. Kessel [1958, p. 45] cites the case of a doctor who acted as an expert witness in California, only to find himself barred from the staff of every hospital in that State. In recent years doctors have been less willing to go to such extremes.

III. Controlling Hospitals

By the 1930s medical care was becoming more and more expensive as it became increasingly dependent on capital investment in equipment and facilities. The result was a growth in the importance of hospitals to provide the new technology and insurance companies to finance its rising cost. Hospitals and insurance companies posed a threat to the power of the organised medical profession, a threat which doctors sought to neutralise. (Insurance companies are discussed in the next Section.)

From the earliest days, the organised medical profession has preferred hospitals to be controlled by self-governing medical staffs, rather than by boards of non-physicians. To prevent hospitals from controlling doctors' fees, doctors also insisted that patients should receive separate bills for physicians' services and hospital accommodation charges.

Medical Profession's Influence over Hospital Management

The AMA's control of medical training has also been used to neutralise the potential power of lay hospital boards of management. Under state laws doctors are required to undergo a period of hospital service before they can be licensed. This year of hospital training, traditionally called an 'internship', had to be undergone in an approved hospital. Interns (first-year graduate trainees) and residents (medical graduates in their second and subsequent years) play an important part in the economics of hospitals, because they can be paid lower salaries. Approval for training is therefore keenly sought and this has put hospitals at the mercy of the AMA which until recently controlled the accreditation of internships and residencies within hospitals. Since 1981 the AMA has shared control of graduate medical education with other organisations through the Accreditation Council for Graduate Medical Education.

Organised medicine has also controlled the general accreditation of hospitals, through the Joint Commission on Accreditation of Hospitals (JCAH), a physician-dominated body made up of representatives from the American College of Physicians, the American College of Sur-

20

geons, the American Dental Association, the AMA and the American Hospital Association (AHA). This control of hospital accreditation was used to discourage competition. For many years, the AMA required hospitals to abide by the 1934 Mundt resolution, which laid down that all hospital staff must be members of the local county medical society. This requirement further enhanced the already considerable power of these local associations. In effect, county medical societies had the power partially to withdraw medical licences, because a doctor cut off from the hospitals would be very limited in the services he could provide [Kessel, 1958, p. 32]. As a result, the organised profession has been able to maintain a solid front against hospital boards which might otherwise have resisted the wishes of their medical staffs. Such boards found themselves threatened with the possibility that every doctor with admitting privileges would send his patients to other hospitals.

Organised medicine has continued to seek to control hospital policy by boycotts and other means. Until 1979 the American Society of Anesthesiologists imposed restrictions on doctors who chose to work for hospitals for a salary. And in 1981 doctors in Brownfield, Texas, threatened to boycott the local hospital's emergency room unless the hospital stopped recruiting outside physicians on terms considered unacceptable by local doctors. Both cases were the subject of FTC intervention, which is discussed in Section VII.

IV. Impeding Insurers

As the cost of medical care increased and hospitals began to play a larger role in the inter-war years, so it became more difficult to finance health outlays by household budgetting and therefore more necessary for individuals to finance health expenditures by insurance. There are two basic methods of health insurance:

(i) cash *indemnity** or reimbursement plans, under which the patient claims a cash benefit in order to meet medical bills, usually actual expenses up to a prescribed limit; and

(ii) *non-indemnity** or *service plans,** under which the insurer provides in kind the level of medical service laid down in the contract. In some variants, payment goes direct from the third-party insurer to the provider; and in others the roles of insurer and provider are integrated.

From the early years of the insurance industry, the organised medical profession sought to prevent insurers from exercising any control over medical practice. The profession adopted three main anti-competitive tactics:

(a) it set out to eliminate competition by establishing producer-controlled insurance plans (Blue Cross and Blue Shield) intent on dominating the industry;

(b) it fought the efforts of other insurers to contain costs;

(c) it vigorously opposed the development of service plans, and especially integrated or pre-payment plans, now called health maintenance organisations (HMOs).

Blue Cross and Blue Shield

By the early years of this century voluntary health insurance had begun to emerge. There are four main types:

---

(1) Hospital expense insurance, covering hospital accommodation charges, emerged first in the 1880s.

(2) Surgical insurance benefit, covering surgeons' and anaesthetists' fees, developed next in 1903.

(3) Medical benefit, embracing non-surgical physicians' fees, followed in 1910.

(4) 'Major medical expense' insurance, offering protection against unusually large medical expenses, came along much later – in the 1950s [Dickerson, 1959, pp. 111, 145].

As health insurance developed rapidly in the 1930s, largely in response to consumer demand, the industry quickly began to be dominated by hospitals and physicians. The initial impetus for Blue Cross hospital expense insurance plans came from groups of employees. Probably the first were a group of Dallas school teachers who tried to organise hospital insurance for themselves in 1929. The result was the Baylor University Hospital Plan, which soon attracted national attention. The group insurance movement received considerable encouragement from the publication in 1932 of the report of the Committee on the Costs of Medical Care, which carried out a major five-year study. It favoured service plans and recommended that medical services should be furnished largely by organised groups of medical personnel, based on a hospital, though it emphasised that fee-for-service medicine should continue unscathed for those who wanted it [Rayack, p. 147]. The AMA was violently hostile and its journal supported the minority report, produced by nine members of the 48-strong committee, dismissing the expenditure of almost a million dollars 'with mingled amusement and regret'. The editorial continued: 'A coloured boy spent a dollar taking twenty rides on the merry-go-round. When he got off, his old mammy said: "Boy, you spent yo' money but where you been?"'.

In the same editorial, group insurance plans organised around hospitals were denounced as 'medical soviets'. The general practitioner, it said, should be restored to 'the central place in medical practice'. In the journal's estimate, 'more than 80 per cent of all the ailments for which people seek medical aid can be treated most cheaply and most satisfactorily by a family physician with what he can carry in a hand-bag'. 'The alignment', concluded the editorial, 'is clear – on the one side the forces representing the great foundations, public health officialdom, social theory – even socialism and communism – inciting to revolution; on the other side, the organised medical profession of this country urging an orderly evolution guided by controlled experimentation . . .'[1]

The *Journal of the American Medical Association* made no secret of the reasons for its opposition: 'One of the chief menaces' of group insurance plans was the 'incitement to solicitation for patients and competitive underbidding'. Such 'half-baked' schemes, insisted another editorial,

'are fraught with danger in placing hospitals on a competitive basis for patients, offering service at prices lower than warranted with subsequent skimping of the service, and, most serious of all, disruption of medical organisation and of the whole institution of medicine'.[2]

Attack on Voluntary Group Insurance

During 1932 and 1933 the AMA published a number of studies emphasising the 'defects' of voluntary group insurance. Their overriding concern was to limit the growth of competition, and to prevent control of medical practice from slipping into the hands of third-party insurers. A report drawn up by the director of the AMA's Bureau of Medical Economics identified 15 defects of voluntary group hospital insurance. The first was that

'such a plan . . . creates a division within the hospital field and the medical profession, and, . . . by creating an artificial monopoly through salesmanship and compulsion by employers is able to exert "unfair competition" on those hospitals outside the schemes. This situation encourages the formation of rival groups and such undesirable forms of commercial competition as solicitation, underbidding and consequent deterioration of service'.

The second defect was even more revealing: 'All such plans tend to lessen the control of county medical societies over medical practice – while at the same time it increases the influence of lay commercial interests'. Defect number six was equally explicit:

'The moment the sphere of commercial competition is permitted to invade

---

[1] *JAMA*, Vol. 99, 1932, pp. 1,950-52.
[2] *JAMA*, Vol. 100, 1933, p. 973.

the organisation, direction and marketing of medical services . . . rival schemes fight for survival by lowering payments for professional services'.

As Rayack comments:

'Clearly, what was involved was a question of medical economics rather than medical "ethics", though the two are often synonymous in the jargon of organised medicine' [Rayack, 1967, pp. 153, 160].

The American Hospital Association (AHA) disagreed with the AMA and, in the hope of maintaining the revenues of hospitals struggling amidst the Great Depression, gave strong encouragement to the organisation of hospital insurance plans from 1933. It formulated a set of principles to guide the schemes being set up all over the country. Group hospital cover was to be non-profit, covering hospital costs only, not doctors' charges. Free choice of doctor or hospital was unchanged, and each plan must be economically sound. But the AHA also sought to discourage competition, urging that advertising should be conducted in a 'co-operative spirit and dignified manner', aimed at selling the plan as a whole and not individual hospital services. In 1936 the AHA began formally to award the right to use the Blue Cross symbol to plans that met these criteria [Dickerson, 1959, pp. 112-13; Rayack, 1967, p. 158]. Blue Cross schemes were usually based on retrospective reimbursement of costs, enabling hospitals to cover their costs, whatever they turned out to be. The typical Blue Cross plan was set up under special state legislation, and was usually supervised by the state insurance department. Normally the self-perpetuating boards of directors comprised hospital representatives, physicians, and members of the public, with the producer dominant.

By 1934 a division of opinion about hospital insurance was emerging within the medical profession. The American College of Surgeons had come out in favour, as had the AMA-affiliated Michigan State Medical Society. Under pressure, the AMA relented slightly, drawing up 10 principles to which voluntary insurance schemes should conform. The first principle gave the game away:

'*All features* of medical service in any method of medical practice *should be under the control of the medical profession.* No other body or individual is legally or educationally equipped to exercise such control' (my italics).

Principle 10 required that 'There should be no restrictions on treatment or prescribing not formulated and enforced by the organised medical profession' [Rayack, pp. 164-5]. Voluntary hospital insurance grew rapidly from 2,000 subscribers in 1933 to 600,000 in 1937, when the AMA was forced reluctantly to accept it.

Medical Opposition to Blue Shield Breaks Down

The next step was the appearance of Blue Shield insurance plans covering the cost of physicians' services. After developing first in California and Michigan in 1939, growth was slow due to a lack of support from most local medical societies, but by 1943 they had 965,000 members, compared with 10 million in hospital plans [Rayack, p. 178; Dickerson, p. 145]. By 1942 the AMA had come reluctantly to accept Blue Shield, but it remained half-hearted until a few years later, when it feared that the Truman administration was about to impose compulsory national insurance on the profession.

Insurance grew rapidly after the war. In 1940, 12 million people (10 per cent of the population) had some form of private health insurance, rising to 77 million in 1950, 122 million in 1960, and 192 million by 1983. The US Bureau of Census estimated that in the fourth quarter of 1983, 85 per cent of the population was covered by either government or private insurance, with 75 per cent of the population covered by private insurance [HIAA, 1985, p. 9]. By 1950 Blue Cross and Blue Shield dominated the insurance market. In that year the 'Blues' sold 51 per cent of all hospital and medical insurance [HIAA, 1985].

Blue Shield plans initially offered service coverage for the lower-paid patient, and cash indemnity to the higher-paid, thus enabling doctors to continue to charge better-off patients fees higher than the insured figure [Hyde et al., p. 984]. Later, a system of 'usual, customary, and reasonable' fees emerged to avoid price competition. Like Blue Cross, Blue Shield plans were established under special state laws and supervised by state insurance departments. The AMA required that they be sponsored by the state or county medical society, under the control of physicians without any third-party involvement, and allow free choice of doctor. Doctors had to be able to set fees in accordance with income and in a manner that was 'mutually satisfactory' [Rayack, p. 51].

Until the early 1970s Blue Cross and Blue Shield were dominated by producer interests. In 1959, 51 per cent of Blue Cross board members were hospital trustees and administrators and a further 17 per cent were doctors and representatives of medical societies. In the early 1960s, 61 per cent of Blue Shield board members were physicians [Goodman and Musgrave, 1985, p. 3]. This producer control of Blue Cross and Blue Shield was significant because it enabled the organised medical profession to exercise a very strong influence over the rest of the insurance market. In particular, it was able to establish the principle that insurers should not interfere with medical judgements, regardless of the implications for cost. Thus, the health insurance industry was dominated by organisations which were concerned to see that producers received the financial returns they sought. Blue Cross, in particular, existed largely to keep hospitals solvent. The usual pressure from insurers to limit costs was therefore missing. By the early 1970s, however, Blue Cross and Blue Shield were beginning to lose market share to cheaper commercial insurance companies which began to adopt a more adversarial role towards the medical profession. In 1972 Blue Cross took the AHA symbol off its logo, and subsequently both Blue Cross and Blue Shield adopted an increasingly critical attitude towards medical fees.

Limiting Cost-Containment by Insurers

Examination of the insurance industry in similar fields like accident, motor or fire insurance shows how insurance companies try to contain costs. Garages in the business of repairing accident-damaged cars find that motor insurance companies are often hard taskmasters, laying down maximum charges, double-checking work estimates, and scrutinising claims. Fire insurance companies treat builders in much the same way. In a competitive industry, this helps to keep premiums lower for the consumer. Until recently economic analysis of health insurance has shown that the industry has not functioned in this manner. The conclusion has frequently been drawn that health insurance is fatally flawed and incapable of containing costs. Section VIII examines recent efforts by insurers to contain costs, but first we must ask why health insurers have not operated in the same manner as other insurers, even when the same company supplied motor, fire or accident insurance as well as health cover.

Study of recent history indicates that they once did. In some states, such as Oregon and Washington, the health insurance industry was well developed by the early years of the century. Doctors were warned

about unnecessary surgery, asked to justify hospitalisation, and had
their bills checked. This supervision did not become general because
organised medicine objected strongly and used a variety of tactics
to stop insurers functioning in a cost-conscious manner.

Goldberg and Greenberg found in Oregon in the 1930s and 1940s
that the insurance market was sufficiently competitive to generate
spontaneous efforts at cost control. Early this century in Oregon insurers, locally called hospital associations, developed to cater for employees in the timber, railroad and mining industries. They were
initiated by physicians but later some were run by lay persons. Some
ran their own hospitals, whilst others used the community hospitals.
The employer and the employee jointly paid a fixed periodic fee and
the hospital association contracted to supply all necessary medical
care. They were profit-making associations, employing some doctors
full-time and others part-time.

The hospital associations usually insisted that no patient be admitted
to hospital (except in emergencies) without the advance approval of
the insurer. Unless treatment orders or tickets had been issued in
advance by the insurer, no bills would be paid. Similarly, no surgery
could be performed without first obtaining a second opinion. This
acted as a safeguard for the patient against unnecessary surgical intervention [Goldberg and Greenberg, 1977a, p. 51]. Doctors resented such
insurance companies, but acquiesced because payment was guaranteed,
a factor of special importance during the depression years.

Until 1941 county medical societies had tried to fight the hospital
associations by setting up their own local pre-payment plans and
expelling doctors involved in 'contract practice'. But they were not
opposed to contract practice as such, only when it was not under the
control of doctors. The new strategy pursued from 1941 was to
establish an alternative state-wide, physician-controlled insurance
company, the Oregon Physicians Service (OPS), to give doctors the
stability of income they sought without controlling fees and utilisation.
Simultaneously, Oregon's physicians refused to deal with the traditional hospital associations.

The usual procedure of the hospital associations when hospitalisation had been recommended was to issue the patient a ticket signify-
ing that the association would pay the bill direct and in full. After
establishing their own insurance company, doctors refused *en masse* to
accept hospital association tickets. This meant that the patient had to

pay the bill himself and then claim from the insurer. The advantage of advance approval over retrospective claiming was that the amount judged by the insurer to be reasonable was settled in advance of treatment, so the patient could be certain of his outgoings. Without advance approval, if the doctor's bill was higher than the insurance company was willing to pay, the patient had to find the balance.

The doctors' boycott soon turned patients against the hospital associations and they switched in large numbers to the OPS. Faced with a loss of business, the hospital associations knuckled under. They stayed in business, but only on the doctors' terms. Efforts to control unnecessary surgery by advance approval and compulsory second opinions were abandoned, and efforts to contain doctors' fees were brought to an end. The case was brought to trial in 1952, but in a now-notorious ruling the courts perversely accepted as legitimate the actions of Oregon physicians in forcing the hospital associations to abandon their efforts to contain professional fees.[1]

Similar anti-competitive action took place in the 1970s. The AMA succeeded in bringing to heel the giant life insurance company Aetna, with around 12 million health policy-holders. It was Aetna's policy that where the doctor's fee exceeded prevailing rates and the doctor and patient could not amicably settle the matter, the company would pay the legal expenses of a patient who was sued by a doctor for non-payment of the outstanding balance. The AMA convention in June 1972 resolved that 'the medical profession will not condone or tolerate action on the part of any third party that would encourage . . . litigation' in fee disputes. A month later a doctor in Florida (successfully) sued an Aetna policy-holder, whose legal fees were paid by Aetna [Rosenberg, 1972]. Doctors were enraged by Aetna's attitude. One doctor suggested in a letter to *Medical Economics* that doctors should refuse to carry out life insurance medical examinations for Aetna, and another suggested that all Aetna patients be boycotted [Goldberg and Greenberg, pp. 63-4]. Under pressure, Aetna backed down and agreed to discontinue its practice of offering to pay patients' legal expenses, and to submit future disputes about fees to a review committee made up of doctors. In practice Aetna abandoned its efforts to contain costs on behalf of policy-holders.

---

[1] *United States* v. *Oregon Medical Society*, 343 US 326 (1952).

Limiting Alternatives to Fee-for-Service

The third tactic of the AMA was to oppose *non-indemnity plans*,* and especially pre-paid group schemes under which the roles of the insurer and the provider were integrated. Now called health maintenance organisations (HMOs), such schemes receive fixed monthly premiums and in return agree to provide specified medical services, when required. HMO premiums naturally reflect age, the services covered in the agreement, family size, and so on, but do not vary with income, so that it was not possible for doctors to continue the custom of charging wealthier patients higher fees.

Traditionally, opposition to HMOs took two main forms: (a) using sanctions to drive existing HMOs out of existence; and (b) seeking legislation in the states to prevent the foundation of new organisations. The general attitude taken by organised medicine was that it was unethical for a physician to sign a contract with any third party where there was competitive bidding or when the payment was considered to be less than the prevailing norm. The AMA also opposed any doctor accepting employment at a salary for any non-medical organisation (including hospitals run by lay boards or committees). In some states doctors were able to secure laws prohibiting physicians from offering their services to the public whilst in the employment of any corporation. The 'corporate practice of medicine' was ostensibly prohibited to stop hospitals or other organisations profiting from the doctor's services.

In reality, such laws were often aimed at HMOs. Legal restrictions against HMOs were achieved in many states. In 1954 at least 20 states had laws intended to discriminate against HMOs and in favour of fee-for-service medicine [Kessel, 1958, pp. 41-2]. The federal HMO Act of 1973 pre-empted state laws for federally-qualified HMOs, but in the late-1970s the Federal Trade Commission was still concerned, and questioned whether the ban on the corporate practice of medicine was necessary to maintain high quality and to protect the public [FTC, 1981a, p. 97].

Laws regulating insurers have also been used subtly to discriminate against HMOs. For instance, the free choice statute of the State of Utah says 'that the right of any person to exercise full freedom of

---

*Glossary, p. 114.

choice in the selection of a duly licensed [provider] shall not be re-stricted' [in Gibson and Reiss, 1983, p. 254]. Such so-called freedom-of-choice statutes have often been interpreted as outlawing the ap-proved panels of doctors around which HMOs are built. HMOs are of service to the consumer precisely because they are based on approved panels of doctors, selected according to their willingness to accept conditions attractive to consumers, such as their ability to supply good quality service at a competitive price. Without the freedom to exclude inefficient doctors, HMOs could not function.

Private professional campaigns to discriminate against HMOs oc-curred across America, affecting numerous organisations. One cel-ebrated case, the Community Hospital-Clinic of Elk City, Oklahoma, was founded by the Farmers Union Hospital Association (FUHA) in 1929. It was a consumer co-operative in which the members owned the hospital and paid the staff fixed salaries. Because medical care was supplied on a pre-paid basis the county medical society tried to drive it out of existence during the first 20 years of its life. Dr Michael Shadid, the first medical director of the hospital, was their chief target. Because he had been a respected member of the medical society for 20 years he could not be expelled, but the county medical society was so deter-mined to get rid of him that it dissolved itself for six months and then re-organised a new county medical society without him. All other hospital-clinic doctors were barred from the county medical society and therefore from the state society and the AMA. In addition, the doctors sought the enactment of legislation that would have outlawed the hospital-clinic. It survived, however, and in 1950 the FUHA took the county medical society to court, charging it with restraint of trade. An out-of-court settlement was reached and sanctions against the hospital-clinic were withdrawn [Rayack, pp. 180-1].

It was not until 1982 that the Supreme Court ordered the AMA to end its support for systematic discrimination against HMOs.

V. Obstructing Auxiliaries

As medical incomes grew in the 1950s because of the restriction of supply there were pressures for less expensive personnel to take on some of the doctors' duties. The use of non-physicians has expanded fast, particularly physiotherapists, occupational therapists, nurses and nurse-midwives. In 1900 there was one doctor for every other health worker. By the early 1960s the ratio was nearly 1:4½ [Rayack, p. 60]. As a result of federal subsidies, this trend accelerated during the 1970s (Section VI) and by 1981 the AMA thought the ratio could be as high as 1:20 [Campion, 1984, p. 456].

FTC Steps in to Help Medical Auxiliaries

The reaction of the AMA has generally been to try to limit the competitive potential of other health-care professionals. Using their control of access to hospitals and medical *malpractice insurance** and their control of physician-dominated Blue Shield plans, doctors have discriminated against colleagues who worked with competing professionals like nurse-midwives. This strategy continued virtually unchecked until the FTC took a stand against it in the late 1970s.

Until the 1970s there were also several severe legal limitations on the roles that could be played by paramedical personnel. Typically, medical practice statutes laid down that

'a person who in any way performs, offers to perform, or holds himself out to the public as performing specific functions – e.g., diagnosing, treating, operating or prescribing for a disease, ailment, pain, or condition – must be licensed as a physician'.

This severely limited competition, but during the 1970s most states began to modify their laws [Goodman, 1980, pp. 40–41]. By 1975 at least 41 had enacted statutes allowing physicians to delegate to physicians' assistants or nurses, though this was a case of law following reality, for it had long been commonplace for nurses to carry out tasks which were legally the exclusive preserve of licensed physicians,

---

*Glossary, p. 113.

such as injections, blood tests, taking temperatures and catheterisation [Rayack, 1967, p. 127]. Nevertheless, the American Nurses Association, representing 170,000 nurses, continues to complain about the disabilities imposed on nurses by regulators in some states. In Alabama in 1982, for example, the board of medical examiners proposed guidelines which would have prevented nurses from functioning at all without a physician present. And in Arkansas the board of medicine was attempting to limit to two the number of nurses a physician could employ or work with at any one time [ANA, 1982, p. 436].

State laws still prescribe the scope of each health occupation, with most states having a licensing board for every health profession. California, for instance, has 11 allied health-care profession boards. Some, like Michigan, have a co-ordinating agency to avoid conflicts of interest [Gibson and Reiss, 1983, p. 255]. The boards interpret and enforce the statutes governing the scope of practice of each occupation. Many such laws are vague, thus giving licensing boards considerable arbitrary power. As a result, occupational relationships are gradually changing at the expense of orthodox medicine.

State insurance law has also restricted competition. Some states have 'freedom-of-choice statutes' laying down that health insurers must cover non-physicians' services, but at the same time they also stipulate that insurers must pay physicians and non-physicians the same fee for like services. This places a barrier in the path of non-physicians who might otherwise offer cheaper alternatives.

Access to hospitals has often been used to obstruct non-physicians who offer popular alternatives. Hospital doctors have been particularly hostile to nurse-midwives. At the Washington Hospital Center, for instance, obstetricians denied hospital privileges to three nurse-midwives who were well respected by patients. Similarly, hospital privileges were denied to nurse-midwives at the Vanderbilt University Hospital [ANA, 1982, p. 436].

Physician-dominated Blue Shield insurance plans have also been used to narrow the market opportunities of competing professionals. In *Virginia Academy of Clinical Psychologists* v. *Blue Shield*, the courts held that Blue Shield's discrimination against non-physician psychotherapists violated the Sherman Act [Havighurst, 1983, p. 309]. Similarly, physician-controlled malpractice insurance companies have been used as weapons. In 1983 a consent order was accepted by the State Volunteer Mutual Insurance Company, a physician-owned medical malpractice insurance firm, not to discriminate against physicians who supervised self-employed nurse-midwives. The insurance company had cancelled the insurance cover of some doctors who worked with nurse-midwives, but this was found to be a boycott which contravened antitrust law.[1]

Despite the AMA's hostility, alternative medicine has expanded rapidly, along with the 'allied' health-care professions. Osteopaths, chiropractors and optometrists were once attacked by the AMA as 'cultists'. All commentators readily concede that the AMA has done much good by attacking and exposing quacks and fraudsters, but its efforts have consistently overflowed into anti-competitive attacks on legitimate and successful alternatives. Osteopaths and chiropractors have achieved legal recognition in all states and enjoy wide public confidence. The number of chiropractors, for instance, despite being classified as 'cultist', more than doubled between 1939 and 1960, when the number of doctors grew by only a third [Rayack, p. 127].

*   *   *

The Evidence So Far

In the Introduction, three main 'market failures' were identified: professional monopoly power, consumer ignorance, and moral hazard. So far in Part 1 we have seen how organised medicine conducted itself until the mid-1970s. Until that time doctors did indeed wield considerable monopoly power. The key to this power was control of the number of doctors in active practice achieved by limiting the number of graduates from medical schools. It proved possible to limit numbers in medical schools because the AMA was able to convince state medical examining boards to recognise only the qualifications of AMA-approved medical schools. Medical examining boards, established in each state ostensibly to protect the consumer, were dominated by the medical profession. The basis of AMA power was therefore the recognition that professional self-regulation was an acceptable method of regulating medical practice.

The evidence so far presented is of a self-seeking medical profession, but, as one recent study found, organised medicine is not solely a

---

[1] FTC, *Annual Report*, 1983, p. 25.

'monopolistic guild'. An important basis of its authority was 'lay deference' [Starr, 1982, p. 144]. This was in part a consequence of the AMA linking its selfish interests with 'good causes'. Early this century, for instance, there were a number of 'degree mills' which churned out doctors after four weeks training armed with virtually worthless paper qualifications. Doctors rightly exposed them, but urged upon state regulators a solution which played into the hands of the profession. The AMA also did much good in the early years of the century by drawing attention to fraudulent medicines, such as William Radam's Microbe Killer, a product which exploited public misunderstanding of the discoveries of Pasteur [Starr, 1982, p. 128]. This campaigning raised the AMA in public esteem, but the AMA was quick to exploit its public standing to extract from governments concessions favourable to the material self-interest of doctors.

In addition, the AMA used a variety of subtle and not-so-subtle private sanctions to discourage competition. They denied cost-cutting doctors access to a number of vital facilities, such as hospital privileges, specialist qualifications, malpractice insurance and even ordinary health insurance plans. They similarly discriminated against non-physicians. The evidence also suggests that consumer ignorance has been manipulated by the medical profession, especially by restricting advertising.

Finally, Part 1 has shown that the failure of third-party insurers to contain costs has been partly a consequence of efforts by organised medicine to monopolise health decision-making. So far, the analysis suggests that the chief 'market failures' are not inherent in the market. We must now examine the evidence of more recent developments before judging how far professionally-inspired obstacles to effective competition can be removed.

PART 2

The Emergence of Competition

VI. Breakdown of Consensus

Concern about the escalating cost of health care was mounting throughout the 1970s. Year by year an ever-rising proportion of national income was consumed by the health industry. In 1950 health care absorbed 4·4 per cent of GNP, in 1970 it had risen to 7·5 per cent, in 1980 it reached 9·4 per cent, and by 1982, 10·5 per cent. Since then the figure has been nudging 11 per cent [HIAA, 1985, p. 45].

The federally-funded *Medicare** and *Medicaid** programmes played a major part in causing these rising costs. From just over one billion dollars spent on Medicare benefits in 1966, the cost rose to 7·1 billion in 1970, 15·6 billion in 1975 and 48·1 billion in 1982 [HIAA, 1985, p. 34]. From 1950 until 1965, the last year before Medicare and Medicaid began, federal, state and local governments funded about a quarter of all US health expenditures. In 1974 the figure reached 40 per cent, and in 1983 it was around 42 per cent [HIAA, 1985, p. 32]. Health-care expenditure has consumed an ever-increasing proportion of the total federal budget. In 1963, 4 per cent of the federal budget was devoted to health care. By 1981 the figure was 13 per cent. As costs rose remedial action became more and more necessary.

Unsuccessful Attempts to Control Health Costs by Regulation

Until the late 1970s, as Americans grappled with rapidly escalating health costs, the vast majority of health experts assumed that government regulation of hospital prices and the limitation of hospital building through state planning agencies were the answer. It was commonly assumed that it was just a matter of time until a compulsory national health insurance scheme was enacted.

Certificate-of-need (CON) reviews of hospital construction plans were first introduced in Maryland in 1968, with other states soon following. Under the 1974 Health Planning and Resources Act, states were required to enact CON laws if they wished to continue receiving federal subsidies, and by 1982 all states except Louisiana had introduced them. In the early years of CON reviews virtually all plans to

*Glossary, p. 114.

establish new health facilities or to add to existing institutions were subject to regulation. Usually regulatory agencies reviewed all proposed expenditures in excess of $100,000 or $150,000, depending on the state. But by the early 1980s confidence in the efficacy of such programmes had diminished. From 1981 only planned expenditures in excess of $500,000 were covered. Definitions of 'need' varied from place to place, as did the make-up of the regulating agency. Generally this type of restriction of entry was liked by existing suppliers because it gave them the chance to stifle competition at birth by arguing that there would be 'duplication', but the effect of CON laws on total hospital expenditure was minimal [Joskow, 1981, p. 241].

In an effort to control Medicare and Medicaid outlays, professional standards review organisations (PSROs) were introduced in 1972 by the Department of Health, Education and Welfare (HEW) (now the Department of Health and Human Services). Hospital records were reviewed case-by-case and contrasted with 'standard' patterns of usage, including admission rates, length of stay, and diagnostic and treatment régimes. Hospitals that could not explain deviations from standard usage profiles could be denied Medicare and Medicaid payments. A review of the system carried out by HEW in 1977 found from a study of 172 PSROs between 1974 and 1976 that they made little impact on *utilisation rates*.* Indeed the cost of the PSRO reviews exceeded any savings [Zeckhauser and Zook, 1981, p. 93]. Not all the evidence has been as negative, but generally there is little to suggest that PSROs have been effective.

The extent of federal involvement in health planning had grown steadily during the 1960s through the Regional Medical Programmes and the Comprehensive Health Planning Act of 1966. But in 1974 the National Planning and Resources Development Act introduced extensive federal control of planning. At the head of the new hierarchy was the Secretary of HEW, then came a national advisory council, then state planning agencies, and finally 204 local Health Systems Agencies (HSAs). They were largely ineffective. A report by the Government Accounting Office found that they tended to set goals that were too vague and sometimes too ambitious. By 1981 the programme had few defenders, and from that year the Reagan administration began to phase out its funding.

---

*Glossary (under 'Utilisation Review'), p. 115.

No Consensus for More Regulation

When the Carter administration's cost-containment legislation was finally defeated in 1979, it became clear that there was no Congressional consensus for still more regulation of health care. By then Americans had 15 years' experience of Medicare and Medicaid behind them, and several years' experience of health planning through HSAs and investment control through CON reviews. None of these inspired confidence in regulation.

Thus, the lack of a consensus for additional regulation pre-dates the Reagan administration. Indeed, the poor results of earlier regulatory experiments contributed to the public mood that made possible his election on an anti-regulation platform. Yet, despite the rhetoric of the Reagan administration, it has not pursued a consistently pro-competitive strategy in health. By refusing to support regulatory schemes brought before Congress, it has nevertheless sent the clear message to health-care providers and insurers: 'You are on your own'. The private sector was galvanised into action, especially employers, who play a vital role in US health care. Around 85 per cent of all private health insurance premiums are paid by group insurance schemes, chiefly because the IRS tax code has since 1954 given employer group health-benefit plans tax-free status.

Escalating Costs to Employers of Health Insurance Schemes

Until recently the tax subsidisation of employer health insurance schemes has discouraged employers from taking the cost-conscious view of health care that they take of every other aspect of their corporate affairs. If an employer gives a member of staff a $1,000 pay rise then he and the employee could pay taxes of between 40 and 50 per cent, but if he gives the employee $1,000 in health benefits no tax is paid. This has made both employer and employee unusually tolerant of cost escalation.

In the late 1970s, however, enormous increases in premiums began to bring a change of heart. From 1982 price escalation was particularly sharp as a result of the reform of Medicare by the Tax Equity and Fiscal Responsibility Act (TEFRA), the first significant effort to tighten Medicare payments to hospitals. In 1983 the Medicare prospective payment system (PPS) came into effect, based on 467 *Diagnosis Related*

*Groups** (DRGs). It had a dramatic impact on hospital finances. Previously, hospitals had charged Medicare more or less whatever they pleased. Henceforward, they would get a fixed sum per DRG – so much for an appendectomy, a hysterectomy, and so on. When hospitals reacted by shifting their costs onto their non-Medicare customers, employers, who were already facing crippling medical costs, bore the brunt.

According to the US Chamber of Commerce, between 1977 and 1983 employer health-care costs increased from 9 per cent of payroll to 11 per cent [Gensheimer, 1985, p. 55; USCC, 1985, p. i]. A 1983 survey of the *Fortune* 500 industrial companies and the 250 largest non-industrial companies found that health costs amounted to 24 per cent of average after-tax profits. Between 1981 and 1983 the average rate of increase of health insurance premiums was 20 per cent. According to the president of one large corporation, health benefits were the third largest cost element after raw materials and 'straight-time pay' for most manufacturers [Herzlinger and Schwartz, 1985, pp. 69-70]. Since 1960, employer contributions to employee health insurance plans have been doubling every five years. Between 1984 and 1985 costs increased 13 per cent to $104·6 billion.[1] These are real increases, reflected in the growing proportion of GNP they consume. Employer contributions were 1·35 per cent of GNP in 1973, increasing to 2·63 per cent in 1983, and falling back slightly to 2·57 per cent in 1984.[2] Some companies faced huge health bills which threatened their business survival. In 1984 Chrysler spent more than $400 million on health care. Adding to this its Medicare taxes of $22 million and a portion of the health insurance premiums of its suppliers, the total comes to $530 for every car sold – around 10 per cent of its cheaper models. In 1970 the cost per car had been $75.

It was these escalating expenditures which compelled employers, who pay the vast majority of private health insurance premiums, to attempt to contain costs. Hitherto, employer groups had looked to government regulation for assistance. From 1969 to 1974 the Nixon administration had frozen prices under its economic stabilisation programme, and in the mid- to late-1970s further price regulation seemed

---

*Glossary, p. 113.
[1] *Coalition Report*, February 1986, p. 1.
[2] *Coalition Report*, March 1986, p. 1.

just a matter of time. But the failure of government regulation persuaded employers that, if costs were to be contained, they must act alone. By removing the huge distortions of the market caused by open-ended Medicare subsidies, the imposition of hospital price-fixing after the enactment of TEFRA in 1982 still further increased the pressure on employers. Long used to the 'cost-plus' system of charging for their services, under which they could pass on their costs without check to both private and government sectors, hospitals now faced cost-conscious buyers of health care across the board.

The remarkable success of employers, described in Section VIII, would not have been possible but for two partly fortuitous developments. First, during the 1970s there was a huge growth in the supply of medical practitioners. And, secondly, as Section VII considers, the Federal Trade Commission intervened decisively to outlaw professional restrictive practices.

The Growth of Supply

For many years control over the supply of doctors by the organised medical profession was considered by economists to be a classic of its kind. A quarter of a century ago Milton Friedman showed how the profession's stranglehold enabled doctors to reap monopoly gains at the expense of their customers and the community [Friedman, 1962, pp. 149-60]. His account has now been overtaken by events.

(a) Physicians: effect of federal subsidies on supply

Direct federal subsidies for medical students were first made available in 1963 when the Health Professions Educational Assistance Act authorised student loans. Previously, only modest construction grants had been made along with subsidies to medical-school affiliated hospitals. In 1965 the Act was amended to allow improvement grants to be made to medical schools which raised the size of their first-year classes [Campion, p. 240]. By 1968 Medicare and Medicaid as well as the Vietnam War had generated increased demand for doctors' services, and in that year President Johnson declared there was a shortage of about 50,000 doctors. Subsequently, federal money flowed into medical schools at an accelerating rate. In 1960-61 federal aid other than on research had been $43 million. Ten years later it was $322 million, and in 1975-76, $398 million. It peaked at $415 million in 1982-83, before dropping in 1983-84 to $390 million [Campion, p. 243; *JAMA*, Vol. 254, 1985, p. 1,576].

The primary purpose of federal subsidies was to increase significantly the number of active doctors, but they have also been used to try to manipulate the specialty mix in the medical profession – for example, by increasing the number of students in family medicine, general internal medicine or general paediatrics by mid-1978 [AMA, 1984, p. 1,516].

Federal subsidies have increased both the number of medical schools and the number of doctors. Medical schools have grown rapidly since the early 1960s. In 1950 there were 79, and in 1960 still only 86. By 1970 there were 103. Five years later there were 114, and by 1984, 127 [BHPr, 1984, Vol. 1, A-1-1].

During the same period the number of graduates also increased sharply. In 1950 there were 5,600 graduates from medical schools. In 1960 there were 7,100, and in 1970, 8,400. Then came a sharp increase. In 1975, 12,700 students graduated, and five years later, 15,100 [AMA, 1984, p. 1,527]. In 1985, 16,300 were expected to qualify.[1]

The number of active doctors has also grown, particularly during the 1970s. In 1950 there were 209,000 active MDs at a ratio of 134 per 100,000 population. In 1963 there were 276,500 at a ratio of only 146. Ten years later there were 366,400 at 174 per 100,000, and in 1981 485,100 at 210 [BHPr, 1984, Vol. 2, B-1-1]. Numbers are expected to increase, with one estimate anticipating 706,500 active doctors by the year 2000 [BHPr, Vol. 2, B-1-35].

This massive increase has dramatically altered the balance of power between doctor and patient. Some young doctors find it impossible to get established in solo practice and therefore find the alternative of salaried employment by an HMO relatively more attractive. The reluctance to compete, which characterised an earlier generation of doctors, has been significantly eroded amongst the young.

The AMA's continuing anti-competitive activities

The AMA continues, however, to try to maintain as tight a grip as it can. One technique has been to extend the time it takes for a doctor

---

[1] *JAMA*, Vol. 254, 1985, p. 1,553.

to qualify. The length of graduate medical education has been steadily increased. In the early days, one year was the minimum requirement, though two or three years of graduate training quickly became common. By 1982 most specialisms required four years and some seven.[1]

In recent years the AMA has sought to increase its control of postgraduate medical education and continuing medical education in the hope of establishing a single, uniform pattern of training. In the mid-1960s frequent clashes between the specialty societies and the AMA threatened the stability of medical practice. According to C. H. William Ruhe, the staff secretary to the AMA's Council on Medical Education, there was a danger of medicine becoming 'balkanised' [Campion, 1984, p. 444]. In his view, 'There should be a single, overall, authoritative body to determine policy and establish standards for the entire field of medical education'. Throughout the 1970s the AMA fought for such a body to ensure that there was a 'continuum from premedical preparation through the continuing education of the practising physician'. Similarly, medical education ought to be 'intertwined with education for the allied health professions and services'. Without such a continuum there would be 'divergent policies', or, in other words, competition [Campion, p. 445].

(b) Non-physicians: rapid growth of assistants and nurse practitioners

Doctors have not only faced increased competition from fellow physicians; the number of members of other health occupations has also increased sharply. This too has been in part a result of a deliberate federal policy. Federal funding has given particular encouragement to physicians' assistants and nurse practitioners.

Physicians' assistants are, as the name implies, trained health practitioners able to provide clinical services under the supervision of a physician. They usually train for two years, with the emphasis on practical work [BHPr, 1984, A-2-5]. Many physicians' assistants are former Vietnam war 'medics'. Between 1972 and 1982 the federal government spent $84 million on training and demonstration programmes. Numbers have grown steadily. In 1983 there were 15,100 physicians' assistants, with 12-13,000 in active practice, a 36 per cent increase since 1980 [BHPr, 1984, A-2-4, B-2-2].

---

[1] *JAMA*, Vol. 254, 1985, p. 1,619.

Federal funding has also been used to encourage the emergence of specialised nurses able to act independently of physicians, usually described as nurse practitioners [BHPr, 1984, C-1-10]. In 1984 there were 18,642 registered nurses described as nurse practitioners or nurse-midwives, which was about 1·3 per cent of all registered nurses [HHS, 1984]. About 36 states have amended their laws to permit the new role, though in practice it is recognised in most. Many studies have shown the effectiveness of nurse practitioners. The report of the Graduate Medical Education National Advisory Committee found in 1980 that

'nurse practitioners and nurse midwives can make positive contributions to the health-care system, can enhance patient access to services, decrease cost and provide a broadened range of services' [in BHPr, 1984, C-1-15].

In 1982 there were 449,000 active doctors of medicine (excluding 18,000 osteopaths). Podiatrists, dentists, optomotrists, pharmacists and registered nurses totalled 1,712,120, of whom 1,357,000 were registered nurses. Between 1970 and 1982 the number of MDs increased by 43 per cent whereas nurses increased in number by 80 per cent over the same period [BHPr, 1984, p. 16]. Osteopaths have only enjoyed full practice rights in some states since 1973, though in 1950 the first osteopaths were given unrestricted rights in some hospitals. In that year there were nearly 11,000 active osteopaths. By 1975 there were 14,060, and by 1981, just under 18,000 [BHPr, 1984, B-1-13].

In addition, huge numbers of 'allied health personnel' came on the scene, including dental assistants, dieticians, medical laboratory workers, occupational therapists, physiotherapists, radiologists, speech pathologists, and physicians' assistants. In 1970 these occupations numbered 658,000, increasing to 1,166,000 in 1982, a 76 per cent rise [BHPr, p. 17; and Table B-8-1].

Many health-care occupations have reached an accommodation with the AMA, on the understanding that they have the status of 'allied professionals'. The AMA co-operates with most of these other health occupations in devising their training programmes, with the aim of giving each a niche in the established order. In 1977 it sponsored the Committee on Allied Health Education and Accreditation (CAHEA) to accredit allied health occupation training programmes. In 1982-83 the AMA collaborated with 40 allied health organisations or specialty societies to set standards for 23 allied health-care occupations [AMA, 1984, p. 1,568]. This makes for a rigid division of

labour and a lack of experimentation with alternative forms of provision. But not all 'allied' health workers have complied, with the
physiotherapists a notable exception.

Alternative medicine continues to flourish. Osteopaths have allowed
themselves to be absorbed into the ranks of orthodox medicine, but
the chiropractors have remained independent. In 1986 it was estimated
that there were around 30,000 chiropractors in active practice, up from
14,000 in 1970 [ACA, 1986, p. 25].

Summary

For most of this century the AMA has been able to limit the number
of doctors in active practice through its control of licensing. But it
proved powerless to prevent huge federal subsidies flowing into
medical schools from the late 1960s onwards. Doctors increased in
numbers so sharply that there is now said to be a 'surplus'. The number
of para-medical personnel has also increased rapidly, again partly due
to federal subsidies. Some of these non-physician groups offer cost-
effective alternatives to orthodox medicine and therefore add to the
competitive pressure faced by the orthodox doctor.

VII. Antitrust Action

The FTC Intervenes

In the mid-1970s the Federal Trade Commission began to investigate the regulation of the professions. The chief reason the FTC chose to focus on the medical profession was disclosed by the new chairman, Mr Michael Pertschuk, in 1977. Conscious of the wide public concern about ever-escalating health costs, he suggested that

'one possible way to control the seemingly uncontrollable health sector could be to treat it as a business and make it respond to the same marketplace influences as other American businesses and industries' [in Greenberg (ed)., 1978, p. 12].

There are two grounds for government intervention to promote competition in the supply of professional services:

(i) The 1890 Sherman Act gives the US Department of Justice the power to bring civil or criminal proceedings against parties acting in restraint of competition.

(ii) Under the 1914 Federal Trade Commission Act (section 5), 'unfair methods of competition' are prohibited. The FTC can order producers to terminate any anti-competitive practice through 'cease-and-desist' orders. These can be challenged in the courts. It also issues advisory opinions and consent orders. Under the latter, the FTC and the producer agree that a particular restrictive practice will stop, without the necessity for litigation. The FTC may also make rules governing competition in a particular industry.

Until 1975, the application of these powers to the professions was somewhat uncertain. There was no statutory exemption as in British law, but the professions had long enjoyed *de facto* immunity, in spite of a case in 1943 when the Supreme Court took a very strong line against an American Medical Association (AMA) boycott of a health maintenance organisation (HMO). The AMA claimed that its action was designed to protect patients' interests but this was firmly rejected by the Supreme Court.[1] In 1952, however, another case had muddied the water. In an *obiter dictum* a judge said:

---

[1] *American Medical Association* v. *United States*, 317 US 519 (1943).

'We might observe in passing ... that there are ethical considerations where the historic direct relationship between patient and physician is involved which are quite different than the usual considerations prevailing in ordinary commercial matters. This Court has recognised that forms of competition usual in the business world may be demoralising to the ethical standards of a profession'.[1]

It was not until 1975 that the Supreme Court took a decisive step towards enforcing antitrust law on the professions. The turning-point came in a case directed against advertising restrictions within the legal profession. In *Goldfarb* v. *Virginia State Bar* the Supreme Court firmly rejected the notion that the 'learned professions' enjoyed immunity from anti-trust law.[2]

The Advertising and Contract Practice Bans

The weapons used by the medical profession to stifle competition have often been subtly chosen, so much so that the AMA has been able to deny with a degree of plausibility that it functioned as a cartel.[3] The AMA often argued that it was merely a voluntary association, whose only power was to expel members, a matter of no more consequence than the expulsion of a member from a sporting or social club. But the Supreme Court has been alive to such sophistries. In another context it has noted that 'experience has shown' business honour and social penalties to be 'the more potent and dependable restraints'. And in another case involving price-fixing among estate agents, the Court observed that 'Subtle influences may be just as effective as the threat or use of formal sanctions to hold people in line' [Havighurst, 1983, p. 298]. This has certainly been true of many of the AMA's anti-competitive manoeuvres.

In December 1975, the FTC brought its first case against the medical profession, when it ordered the AMA to desist from enforcing restraints on advertising and to abandon its policy of discriminating against alternative delivery systems like HMOs. In 1980 a final order was issued requiring the AMA to stop interfering with prices charged by its members or characterising as unethical the use of approved

1 *United States* v. *Oregon State Medical Society*, 343 US 326 (1952).

2 421 US 773 (1975).

3 *American Medical Association* v. *FTC*, 638 F.2d 443 (2d Cir. 1980); 452 US 960 (1982).

panels of doctors or the participation of non-physicians in the owner-
ship or management of health-care organisations. After a long legal
battle the FTC order was affirmed by the Supreme Court in 1982.[1]

Under the order, the AMA was prohibited from restricting truthful
advertising, but permitted to police 'false or deceptive' claims made in
advertisements. This concession has been criticised by some academic
observers like Professor Clark Havighurst, a leading authority from
Duke University, who believes it contains a 'potential for unchallenged
harm' by allowing the AMA to keep power which could be used to
'harass and intimidate' other doctors [1983, p. 307]. The FTC order
also prohibited the AMA from anti-competitive interference with
arrangements made for the supply of medical care by any doctor,
whether in a hospital, an HMO, or anywhere else. The Court of
Appeals also prohibited AMA rulings which prevented doctors from
forming partnerships with allied health-care professionals. The FTC
found that these rules impeded the emergence of economically more
efficient forms of practice.[2]

Medical School Accreditation

Section I showed how the AMA has used medical school accreditation
to increase the take-home pay of doctors. This history of abuse led
the FTC to investigate the AMA's role in accreditation, which today is
a function of the Liaison Committee on Medical Education (LCME).
In 1985 six of its 17 members were appointed by the American Association of Medical Colleges and seven by the AMA, with two public
members, one a government representative and one representing
Canadian medical schools.[3] By law the LCME must periodically
petition the federal Office of Education for official recognition. Until
1977 it was required to seek re-authorisation every four years, but in
March of that year the FTC's Bureau of Competition advised the
Office of Education to deny the LCME recognition, arguing that the
AMA's influence over it was incompatible with the public responsi-

---

[1] The AMA appealed in 1980 to the Second Circuit Court of Appeals, arguing that it
had already abandoned the practices complained of, but the Appeals Court upheld the
FTC ruling (638 F.2d 443 (1980)). The Supreme Court heard the AMA's further appeal
in 1982 and tied 4-4, thus affirming the Appeals Court decision (452 US 969 (1982)).

[2] FTC Order in *JAMA*, 27 August 1982, pp. 981-2.

[3] *JAMA*, Vol. 254, 1985, p. 1,619.

bilities of an accrediting agency. At that time, not only did the AMA appoint six of its members, it also contributed half its funding, and directly administered the scheme every other year. According to the Bureau, it was therefore very strongly placed to influence the judgements of the LCME. Greater autonomy was required to avoid this clash of interests. The federal Commissioner of Education did not withdraw recognition, but limited it to two years. Because the huge growth in the number of doctors described in Section VI (pp. 43-44) has swamped the AMA's restrictions, no further action has been found necessary by the FTC.

Interfering with Insurers

The FTC recognised that since insurance coverage weakened or removed the insured person's incentive to contain medical costs, the efforts of insurance companies to limit outlays should not be impeded. To the extent that insurance companies sought to reduce medical expenditures they were acting in pursuit of the consumer's interests. As we have seen, three strategies have been used by doctors to restrict cost-containment by insurers: boycotts against insurers who sought to influence prices or utilisation rates; discrimination against HMOs; and the foundation of physician-controlled insurance plans, like Blue Shield.

Again, doubt remained about the applicability of antitrust law to the professions until the Department of Justice brought an important case in 1978. In *National Society of Professional Engineers* v. *United States*, the professional engineers argued that their code of ethics, which prohibited members from submitting competitive bids, was justified because it prevented competition from generating inferior-quality work. The Supreme Court ruled that there were no exceptions to the Sherman Act. Expressing the majority view, Justice Stevens said:

'The Sherman Act reflects a legislative judgement that ultimately competition will not only produce lower prices, but also better goods and services . . . The assumption that competition is the best method of allocating resources in a free market recognises that all elements of a bargain – quality, service, safety, and durability – and not just the immediate cost, are favourably affected by the free opportunity to select among alternative offers. Even assuming occasional exceptions to the presumed consequences of competition, the statutory policy precludes inquiry into the question whether competition is good or bad.'

This judgement plainly threw doubt on the medical profession's claim that its anti-competitive contrivances were designed to protect the consumer. But until 1982 it was not certain that the courts would apply the same thinking to doctors. Some anti-competitive actions – such as price-fixing, geographical carve-ups, group boycotts, tie-in deals, and allocation agreements – are seen as *per se*, or automatic, violations of the Sherman Act. In other cases the 'rule of reason' may apply. This notion is defined in the FTC enforcement policy on doctor-controlled medical prepayment plans. Generally, concerted activities are illegal only if they unreasonably restrain trade:

> 'Under this "rule of reason", there must be an examination of the purpose for which the parties have entered into the agreement or course of conduct and of the effects that have resulted or are likely to result from their concerted activity. Any pro-competitive effects are weighed against anti-competitive effects in determining whether the restraint, on balance, is unreasonable'.

The focus of the inquiry is whether or not the restraint under investigation promotes or suppresses competition [FTC, 1981b].

The issue came up in a case concerning fixed-fee schedules. Traditionally, doctors have laid down fees and applied sanctions against colleagues who charged less and against insurance companies who paid below AMA rates. In *Arizona* v. *Maricopa County Medical Society*, the Supreme Court held that the establishment of *maximum* fees for medical services was price-fixing, and therefore a *per se* violation of the Sherman Act. The case concerned two physician-controlled 'foundations for medical care' which laid down maximum fees participating doctors could charge when patients were covered by insurers who had accepted the foundations' fee schedules. Even though maximum rather than minimum fees were being controlled, the Court ruled against price-fixing as such, finding that 'Even if a fee schedule is . . . desirable, it is not necessary that the doctors do the price fixing'. Insurers could just as easily do it.[1]

In another case, the FTC accused the Michigan State Medical Society, which represented 80 per cent of the state's doctors, of engaging in an unlawful conspiracy to fix physician fees. For instance, it collected written proxies empowering the society to cancel doctors' arrangements with Blue Cross/Blue Shield and Medicaid if they did

---

[1] 102 S Ct. 2466,2477 (1982).

not accept the society's terms. The Michigan State Medical Society was forbidden by the court to continue this practice and prohibited from negotiating re-imbursement terms on behalf of its members.[1]

The FTC has focussed particularly on the efforts of dentists to deny insurers information on which to base cost control. It issued consent orders to stop the Indiana Federation of Dentists and the Texas Dental Association collectively refusing to submit dental X-ray films requested by insurers.[2] The Texas Dental Association agreed not to interfere with insurance companies' efforts to minimise costs by requesting X-rays to evaluate the treatment planned for policy-holders. The Indiana Federation appealed but the Supreme Court unanimously upheld the FTC ruling.

*Peer review** is another device by which the medical profession has been able to arrogate to itself the power to settle matters about which insurers have a legitimate concern. By insisting that professional peer review committees should be the sole arbiters of disputes between doctors and insurers about fees or utilisation rates, doctors have been able to discourage cost containment. According to Havighurst, the *Maricopa County* case (above, p. 52) outlaws professional demands to have the final say in fee disputes, but an element of doubt remains [1983, p. 312].

Provider Control of Pre-payment Plans

Antitrust law has put a stop to a number of practices which were plainly anti-competitive. A more difficult area is the direct control by doctors of insurance plans like Blue Shield. In the mid-1970s the FTC set out to establish whether the medical profession influenced Blue Cross and Blue Shield insurance plans in such a manner as to modify the normal incentive of the insurance industry to minimise costs. It found that not every case of producers getting together to offer a service could be construed as anti-competitive, and for this reason found it difficult to lay down hard-and-fast rules. It determined, therefore, to proceed on a case-by-case basis, in accordance with the principles laid down in an enforcement policy published in 1981.[3]

Usually, a combination of a relatively small proportion of physicians in a locality in a 'merged' or group arrangement would not raise

---

[1] FTC, *Annual Report*, 1983, p. 49.   [2] FTC, *Annual Report*, 1983, pp. 43,49.
[3] 46 *Federal Register* 48982 (1981).   *Glossary, p. 114.

antitrust concerns. As a rule of thumb, up to 30 per cent of physicians in a locality could be involved. The document distinguishes between group practices, like staff or group model HMOs (below, p. 68) and 'partially integrated' plans like foundations for medical care, independent practice associations (IPAs) and Blue Shield plans. The latter are examined under the 'rule of reason', and the pro- and anti-competitive effects weighed before final judgement is made. However, if a partially-integrated scheme covered two-thirds or more of active physicians in a locality, it would be very likely to be judged anti-competitive. Approved panels of doctors, the document points out, are pro-competitive insofar as they encourage choice between those on the panel and those outside it.

Denying Access to Hospital Privileges

The denial of access to hospital facilities has been a common device used by hospital medical staffs against HMOs or price-cutting physicians. The principle the FTC has asserted is that a hospital can be selective so long as its judgement is not influenced by anti-competitive considerations. Thus, in selecting staff a hospital may take into account professional 'track record', willingness to accept the hospital's preferred salary, or to participate in discounting arrangements with insurers, and so on, but it may not allow its medical staff to deny hospital facilities to physicians because the newcomers will compete with insiders or because they do not conform with professional restrictive practices.

For instance, consent order proceedings were initiated in 1979 to stop doctors of the Pittsburgh Hospital Group denying hospital privileges to colleagues associated with the Forbes Health System HMO.[1] Similarly, medical staffs may not deny hospital facilities to non-physicians like podiatrists (chiropodists), osteopaths, or nurse-midwives [Havighurst, 1983, p. 309].

Mergers and Takeovers

Where it sees a possibility of local market domination, the FTC has intervened to prevent hospital mergers and takeovers. For instance,

---

[1] FTC, *Annual Report*, 1980, p. 52.

American Medical International, a for-profit hospital company, was ordered in 1983 to dispose of a hospital in California because its purchase in 1979 had been an attempt to reduce price and non-price competition.[1]

Conclusion

Antitrust law has been enforced against most of the restrictions identified in Part 1, although some obscurities remain. Specialty certification is still open to abuse by denying entry to newcomers, and the restriction of comparative information persists [Greenberg, 1984]. The American Hospital Association still warns against making direct comparisons between one hospital and another, but, careful to avoid the attentions of the FTC, it advises only that direct comparisons should not be made 'unless they can be measured and substantiated' [AHA, 1977]. Access to PSRO (now PRO) findings is not wholly satisfactory. PRO investigations could be a source of evidence about the competence of doctors and hospital departments which consumers could well find useful. Indeed, access to information about the quality of individual physicians or hospitals is strongly resisted by all providers. Nevertheless, the record of the antitrust enforcement agencies since the mid-1970s has been impressive. Section VIII considers whether the anticipated advantages of competition have emerged in practice.

---

[1] FTC, *Annual Report*, 1983, p. 47.

VIII. Transformation Through Competition

The re-awakening of competition in the US market as the balance of power has shifted in favour of the consumer owes much to the efforts of employers. An early reaction was to form health coalitions, or local business groups, to seek a unified approach to rising medical costs. Between 1978 and 1981, 50 emerged; in 1983 the US Chamber of Commerce listed 103 and, according to the AHA,[1] by 1985 there were 151. A typical example is Dallas, where in the early 1980s a handful of business leaders began by discussing informally their common worries about rising health costs. The outcome was the formation of the Dallas Business Group on Health in 1982. By 1985 it had 32 affiliated companies. Most coalitions are dominated by purchasers, though insurers and providers are frequently represented. By 1984 the AMA, the AHA, and the Health Insurance Association of America (HIAA) each had departments charged with promoting the involvement of insurers or suppliers in the work of the new coalitions.

National Health Coalitions

National groups have also developed. The Washington Business Group on Health was established in 1974, the Business Roundtable founded its Health Initiative in 1981, and the US Chamber of Commerce established its Clearinghouse on Business Coalitions for Health Action in 1982 [Lewin and Associates, 1984, Chapter V].

Some local coalitions have become pressure groups seeking state price-fixing laws, such as in Massachusetts, but most have sought to promote cost-saving reform of benefit plans and to encourage the emergence of new cost-effective delivery systems like HMOs and preferred provider organisations (PPOs). They have frequently sought the co-operation of county medical societies and local hospitals in identifying and re-educating 'rogue' providers. Thus, the Dallas

---

[1] *Hospitals*, 16 December 1985, p. 43.

Business Group on Health co-operates with the local county medical society in identifying doctors who regularly hospitalise their patients more frequently than their colleagues, perhaps ordering hospital stays of 10 days for a given complaint when seven is usually found adequate. There may be good reasons why a doctor does not conform to some standard pattern but, in any event, the Dallas group co-operates with the county medical society to identify 'outliers' and to seek explanations for any deviance. After many years of intransigent hostility to lay interference with the doctor's judgement, many county medical societies are happy to co-operate with such programmes, and the AMA nationally claims it is content to look upon this kind of monitoring as a part of the doctor's education, though they still insist that all final decisions must lie with physicians.

Trend to Self-Insurance

One striking trend has been the shift away from traditional group health insurance to *self-insurance*.* Under the traditional group system each employee group is 'experience-rated' by the insurance company, according to its history of claims. Schemes vary, but generally premiums are calculated by estimating likely benefit payments and adding a proportion for administration and profit. If costs exceed revenue, losses are recouped the following year. If there is a surplus, a dividend may be paid to contributors. The insurer pays claims out of the premium income held.

Self-insurance usually operates as follows. Instead of paying premiums to the insurer who holds them in order to pay claims, the employer agrees to pay an insurer a fixed amount to process claims, but holds the premiums himself in a special account. The insurer provides *administrative services only** (ASO) – that is, he receives the claim forms and pays claims out of the employer's special account. For the employer this improves cash flow and widens the choice of organisations available to process claims. Some companies, for instance, do not use an insurance company at all. They have brought in specialist fund management agencies or third-party administrators (TPAs), of which a number have emerged (over 100 are listed in the *Business Insurance* directory). Some companies have gone further still and opted

---

*Glossary, p. 114.   *Glossary, p. 113.

for *self-administration*,* in which case they can control expenditure on administration directly.

But the trend towards self-insurance is not only a consequence of the desire of employers for increased freedom of action in their dealings with insurers. It is also the result of changes in federal law. In 1974 the Employee Retirement Income Security Act (ERISA), which regulates pension plans for workers in the private sector, enabled employers who provided employee welfare benefits through self-insurance to escape the jurisdiction of state insurance laws.

Under state laws there are three types of insurer: Blue Cross and Blue Shield, the commercial insurers, and the self-insured. The 'Blues' and commercials both face financial and benefit regulation by state insurance departments. This includes controlling initial solvency, reserves, types of investment, and premium rates. Premium taxes of about 2 per cent are usually levied on the commercial insurers, and sometimes on the Blues, though in about half the states premium taxes are not imposed on Blue Cross and Blue Shield. Self-insurers avoid premium taxes and regulation by state insurance departments, and of particular value, they are not bound by state laws mandating certain benefits. In recent years many states have required all insurers to provide mandatory benefits like treatment for alcoholism or drug dependency and mental illness, and this restricts the freedom of employers and employees to devise an insurance package to meet their own needs. As Section V showed, some state laws also forbid price discrimination. Self-insurance enables companies to escape these and similar anti-competitive laws.

The disadvantage of self-insurance is that in a very bad year the employer may find himself facing unexpectedly high losses. A mechanism has emerged to cover this eventuality – the *minimum premium plan** (MPP). The MPP is an arrangement under which companies self-insure up to a ceiling. Usually a company accepts liability up to an agreed monthly or annual maximum. It would hold, say, 90 per cent of premiums and pay the remainder to an insurer to cover catastrophic losses. The employer gains the advantages of self-insurance, including avoidance of state insurance premium taxes on all but the sum paid to the insurer, whilst containing potential losses within acceptable limits.

---

*Glossary, p. 114.   *Glossary, p. 114.

The extent of the shift towards self-insurance has been measured by several surveys. A study of the *Fortune* 500 top industrial companies and the 250 largest non-industrials in 1983 found that 97 per cent had some element of self-funding and 57 per cent were wholly self-funded [Herzlinger and Schwartz, 1985, p. 76]. A survey of mainly large companies conducted by management consultants Towers, Perrin, Forster and Crosby in New York, found that 62 per cent of employers self-funded company health plans in 1985, up from 43 per cent in 1982. In another survey, the Wyatt Co. found that 75 per cent of employers with between 7,501 and 10,000 employees self-funded their health plans, up from 25 per cent in 1980. It is now becoming difficult to find a large company not involved in some way in self-insurance. But small companies are also turning to it. According to the Wyatt survey, 55 per cent of employers with fewer than 500 staff were self-insured in 1984, up from 18 per cent in 1980.[1]

Changes in Market Shares

These developments have brought about changes in the market shares of insurers. According to the US government's Health Care Financing Administration, in 1965 Blue Cross/Blue Shield had 45 per cent of the private insurance market, already reduced from the 1950s, whilst commercial insurers had 48 per cent. Prepaid plans had 2 per cent and self-insured/self-administered schemes, 5 per cent. By 1983 Blue Cross/ Blue Shield were down to a 35 per cent share. Self-insured/self-administered plans had 8 per cent, third-party administrators 3 per cent and prepaid plans 6 per cent. Commercial insurers continued to hold a 48 per cent share, but the nature of their business had changed dramatically. In 1965, 81 per cent of their share was in the form of group policies. By 1983 group plans accounted for only 50 per cent of their business. Minimum premium plans accounted for 29 per cent and administrative services only schemes, 15 per cent. Altogether, self-insurance (including self-administration, TPAs and ASOs) and quasi-self-insurance (MPPs) accounted for 32 per cent of private health insurance in 1983 [Arnett and Trapnell, 1984, pp. 34-5].

The shift to self-insurance does not in itself reduce costs, though it helps by enabling employers to escape premium taxes and state legal

---

[1] *Business Insurance*, 27 January 1986, pp. 3-4.

requirements to provide ever more comprehensive and costly benefits. Above all, employers gain increased flexibility to design tailor-made health packages. They have seized the opportunity offered, on the one hand by self-insurance and on the other by the recent shift in the balance of market power in favour of the purchaser, to demand more cost-conscious health insurance. This has been achieved partly by modifying health plans to increase the extent of cost-sharing with the employee in order to overcome the moral hazard inherent in third-party funding, but, as I will consider below, much has also been achieved by introducing administrative mechanisms that involve no sharing of costs.

Cost-Sharing

Traditional group health plans usually gave employees comprehensive cover, with very little cost-sharing. At each pay round, which in America has generally meant every three years, trade unions or work-force representatives sought to increase health benefits as part of the wage bargain. In a competitive labour market employers were ever anxious to present themselves as 'generous' and readily agreed to more and more extensive health benefits, so long as they could pass on part of the cost to the community through tax subsidisation. The disadvantage of the traditional group scheme was that neither employer nor employee had much regard for what it all cost, and in the end, as we have seen, this led to such rapid cost escalation that for some companies health bills threatened their very survival.

Co-insurance

Remedial action became unavoidable and one obvious measure was to introduce cost-sharing to ensure that individual employees faced an incentive to think about costs whilst continuing to be protected against serious illness. Instead of paying 100 per cent of all or most medical bills, companies introduced or extended *co-insurance*,* whereby the employee usually pays 20 per cent. *Deductibles*,* whereby the employee pays all medical bills up to an agreed sum before cover begins, have also been increased. Traditional group policies often had

---

*Glossary, p. 113.   *Glossary, p. 113.

a small deductible of $50 a year. Employers have sought to increase it to $200 or more. Some employers have introduced individual 'stop-losses' to protect employees who face heavy expenditures in a given year. Rockwell, for instance, places an annual maximum of $500 per person or $1,000 per family on *co-payments.** In some cases these individual stop-losses have been linked to salary. At LTV, a company with 55,000 employees including many in the highly unionised steel industry, the annual deductible is limited to 1 per cent of basic salary, and co-payments are restricted to 2 per cent.

Financial incentives to make low-cost choices are often built into schemes. Co-payments may be waived or reduced if, for example, instead of going into hospital, the patient has surgery in an outpatient department, in the doctor's surgery, or in an ambulatory (day) surgery centre. The first ambulatory surgery centres independent of a hospital emerged in 1970 in Rhode Island and Arizona. They do not have the high overheads of hospitals and because they have no inpatients are usually much cheaper. The use of ambulatory surgery centres saved Blue Cross and Blue Shield of North Carolina $5·3 million in the first half of 1985, and Blue Cross of Philadelphia announced it was distributing to policy-holders $55·9 million in special 'utilisation awards', equivalent to one month's premium each, in recognition of their use of more cost-effective suppliers.[1]

Similarly, financial incentives have been offered to take second opinions when surgery has been recommended. Rockwell, for instance, will pay only 50 per cent of the cost of surgery if no second opinion has been obtained. Second opinions often produce non-confirmation rates of between 25 and 35 per cent.

Flexible spending accounts

Another cost-sharing device is the individual medical expense account, or flexible spending account (FSA). When LTV revised its health plan in 1984 it introduced co-payments and increased its deductible, when previously it had paid 100 per cent of all bills. To preserve the tax-free status previously enjoyed by employees it established FSAs. Staff could pay into their FSA by payroll deduction and withdraw

---

*Glossary, p. 113.

[1] *Consumer Exchange*, January and March 1986.

from it to meet co-payments and deductibles. Such payments are tax free, just as if the company has paid for the health care in the first place. According to a survey of 861 companies carried out by the consulting firm A. S. Hansen, 14 per cent had established a health-care spending account for individuals. Just under one-third made a company contribution.[1] Xerox, for instance, agreed to pay $400 per employee into a personal medical expense account, the amount they had saved by redesigning their health plan. Initially, money not used on co-insurance or deductibles was allowed to accumulate at interest to be taken in cash at the end of the year, though legal changes now prevent this from being done. Flexible spending accounts have been less popular since the Deficit Reduction Act of 1984 required individuals to forfeit the balance remaining in their FSA at the end of the year, instead of taking it as taxable income.

Flexible multiple-choice plans

Several companies have introduced flexible benefits packages in which employees choose between health plans at varying costs. If they choose a cheaper one, they share in the savings. The oldest example of a multiple-choice plan is the Federal Employees Health Benefits Plan, which covers employees of the federal government. Employees receive a fixed dollar subsidy and may choose from among a number of registered alternatives. In a few cases companies have introduced 'cafeteria' plans, offering an array of tax-deductible benefits like pensions as well as health care. Savings made from one plan may be spent on another benefit, though not taken as cash. Some firms have hesitated to develop such plans because of the uncertainty which has surrounded their tax status. The chief advantage for the employer is that in each contract cycle he can agree to contribute a fixed cash sum, whereas in the past employers often agreed to supply a prescribed set of health benefits and then had to go out and buy the previously agreed package in an uncompetitive market. The employee gains flexibility. If he chooses to invest more in a pension than in a health plan he can do so. This is especially helpful to the growing number of families with two wage-earners. Instead of being in two health plans, one partner

---

[1] *Coalition Report*, February 1986, p. 7.

can gain family health cover at his workplace, and the other partner can invest up to the hilt in a pension or other benefit at hers.

Again, LTV is probably typical. It offers its 55,000 staff over a dozen alternatives. The company provides certain 'base benefits', like medical cover and disability benefit, and in addition a variety of others can be obtained from the 'supplemental salary', an earmarked element of salary calculated as a percentage of base earnings and increased with length of service. The employee can choose between additional health benefits, day care, legal services, disability income, life insurance, accident insurance, pension, and alternative forms of capital accumulation, including an in-house company scheme and the federal individual retirement account.[1]

There are a number of studies of the impact of cost-sharing. At one time some economists believed that doctors had sufficient market power to be able to manipulate demand. V. R. Fuchs, for instance, claimed that a 10 per cent increase in the surgeon/population ratio resulted in a 3 per cent increase in surgery [1978, pp. 35-6], and in an older study M. S. Feldstein argued that doctors were able to exercise similar power within the NHS [1967, pp. 196-200, 278-80]. Other studies contradict their conclusions. A huge examination of the effects of cost-sharing on utilisation rates conducted for the US Department of Health and Human Services by the Rand Corporation found that expenditure per person varied according to the extent of cost-sharing Expenditure per person was about half as large in insurance plans without cost-sharing as it was in plans which required 95 per cent co-insurance up to a $1,000 maximum in a year. The study concluded that 'cost-sharing unambiguously reduces expenditure' [Newhouse et al., 1982]. A further study, also conducted by the Rand Corporation, examined the effects of cost-sharing on health status. It contrasted the health of 3,958 patients aged between 14 and 61, some of whom were members of insurance plans requiring cost-sharing and some of whom were not. Patients in cost-sharing plans visited doctors about one-third less frequently and entered hospital about one-third less often. People with poor eyesight and low-income individuals with high blood pressure were slightly better off under 'free' plans, but for the average participant, and regardless of income or initial health condition, no significant effects on their subsequent health were detected [Brook et al.,

---

[1] LTV, *Benefit Planning Kit.*

1983]. Thus, cost-sharing appears to produce a lower use of medical services without impairing health.

Administrative Mechanisms with no Cost-Sharing

Under some plans, second opinions for surgery are compulsory, with the plan paying in full for second and even third opinions. Counselling is also growing, in order to advise employees faced perhaps with a recommendation for 'unnecessary' surgery. Blue Cross and Blue Shield of Illinois and the Zenith company introduced a Medical Services Advice Program in January 1983 for 3,000 staff in Chicago. Employees faced with hospitalisation are invited to talk it over with Zenith's medical adviser. They discuss cheaper or more effective alternatives, but any change is wholly at the patient's discretion. If asked, the medical adviser will also discuss the case with the physician. The Blues plan to extend the scheme. The Teamsters union offers a phone-in and walk-in advice service to 14 branches in New York, New Jersey, and Connecticut. It will recommend reliable and cost-effective providers and arrange referrals, if requested [Lewin and Associates, II, pp. 43-5].

Advance approval or *pre-admission certification** is now frequently required for all recommended hospital stays. When LTV introduced its revised health plan in April 1984, some cost-sharing through pay-related deductibles and co-payments was entailed, but the chief cost-saver was the requirement that all hospital stays must be the subject of advance approval by the insurer. Under the old plan, hospital admissions between January 1982 and March 1984 had taken place at the rate of 154 per 1,000 plan members. Between April 1984 and February 1985 hospital admissions fell to 93, a 40 per cent reduction. On a *per capita* basis, hospital inpatient claims fell by 41 per cent, from $2,021 to $1,196, though there was an additional cost of $275 because of more intensive use of outpatient facilities.[1]

Other insurers have introduced convalescent benefits to encourage people to obtain care outside hospital: home care is a popular alternative, supported by a visiting nurse or a home health agency. Another option is a skilled nursing facility (SNF); and thirdly, for the long-term sick, there is care in a hospice or nursing home.

---

*Glossary, p. 114.   [1] LTV, internal memorandum.

Child birth has been especially affected by pressures to discourage people from staying in hospital. Blue Cross and Blue Shield of Philadelphia encourage mothers to go home after 24 hours, but pay for home nurse visits and homemaker/aide visits. Blue Cross in Rochester, New York, provides three days' home support with homemaker/aide back-up. This costs $70 a day, compared with hospital inpatient fees of $300 a day. Insurers also encourage the use of independent 'birthing' centres in place of hospital maternity wards [Lewin and Associates, 1984, II, p. 28].

The changed attitude towards hospitals is not only the result of a desire to save money. It also reflects a wider determination by people not to have their lives controlled. Pregnant women led the way in refusing to be dictated to in the intensely personal matter of child birth. The home birth movement was a protest at the way in which child birth, an essentially natural act, had been turned into an 'illness' subject to regimentation by professionals. Women demanded to remain at home with their husbands present, often preferring the female midwife to the (mostly male) doctor. Partly in response, specialist 'birthing' centres emerged to provide a home-like atmosphere, with the extra safeguards which are helpful in emergencies. Hospitals, too, had to respond, and now delivery rooms often mimic the home environment with homely wallpaper and soft furnishings, with fathers attending births as a matter of routine. Hospitals are, nonetheless, large institutions which can run only by routine and discipline, and are having difficulty holding their market share.

'Wellness' incentives for subscribers

Both employers and insurers are seeking to encourage subscribers to take better care of themselves. Insurers offer non-smokers' discounts. Blue Cross and Blue Shield plans in Washington and Alaska, Oregon, Minnesota, Virginia, Idaho and Texas have introduced discounts of around 10 per cent for non-smokers.[1] Many employers offer 'wellness' programmes. A survey of 191 organisations in New England by the consulting firm William M. Mercer-Meidinger, found that over 62 per cent were promoting self-help. Some sponsored health education classes and literature, others established facilities to monitor conditions

---

[1] *Consumer Exchange*, November 1985.

like high blood pressure, and some subsidised employee membership in fitness facilities.[1] The 1984 Business Roundtable survey of 122 employer health plans covering 7·5 million employees found that one-third gave new employees physical examinations, and a quarter offered periodic check-ups to all staff. Half provided keep-fit programmes, and many provided employee counselling on alcohol and drug abuse or personal and family problems [Business Roundtable, 1985].

Faced with a huge loss of market share, Blue Cross and Blue Shield have had to change their role significantly. They now actively promote HMOs and PPOs. In addition, most Blue plans offer 'managed care', a traditional indemnity insurance package re-inforced by cost-containment measures. Master Health Plus, introduced by Blue Cross of Massachusetts, is a fairly typical managed-care scheme. Benefits are comprehensive, with limited cost-sharing: a $5 co-payment for visits to the doctor's surgery; a $25 deductible for hospital outpatient procedures; and a $3 charge for generic drugs and $4 for branded medicines. The main savings come from *utilisation review*.* Following the lead of other insurers, pre-admission review of hospital stays has been introduced. Failure to get pre-admission approval (except in emergency) means that the subscriber must pay the first $1,000 of any bill.

During pre-admission review the insurer's representative, usually a registered nurse, judges whether hospitalisation is necessary, or whether outpatient care may be cheaper. The nurse reviewer also tries, where appropriate, to schedule surgery on the day of admission, and to co-ordinate lab tests and X-rays in advance. Pre-admission diagnostic testing is often carried out on a massive scale, and from 1979 Blue Cross and Blue Shield sought to modify hospital practice by discouraging the indiscriminate carrying out of 'admission batteries' of tests such as blood haemoglobin, urine analysis, bio-chemical blood screens, chest X-rays and electrocardiograms. Physicians were urged to order each specific test individually and thus to think carefully about the necessity for each. In some hospitals 'guest rooms' have been introduced at about $25 a night. Patients who can otherwise look after themselves can stay in the guest room before surgery, when this

---

is convenient. This compares with the average local hospital charge of $500 a day.

Mandatory second opinions

Second opinions for surgery have been made mandatory because Blue Cross has found financial incentives to consult a different specialist an insufficient inducement. Blue Cross pays for second and even third opinions, but patients failing to comply must pay the first $1,000 of the hospital bill and all the surgeon's and anaesthetist's charges. Otherwise Blue Cross pays in full.[1] During hospitalisation there is on-site *concurrent review*,* to double check the necessity for diagnostic and surgical procedures carried out in hospital and to avoid unnecessarily long stays. Discharge planning is also a common feature of managed care. Nurse reviewers ensure that physicians do not allow patients to remain in hospital any longer than required, and make arrangements for home care backed by specialist nursing support or other alternatives. This is not only a matter of saving money, it is also in the patient's interest to avoid staying in hospital longer than necessary, for hospitals are the home of virulent infections. In 1983, according to one estimate, nearly 2 million patients contracted new illnesses in hospital, and 96,000 died as a result.

The cost-containment mechanisms built into managed care have achieved very significant savings, though at this early stage the evidence is unsystematic. The Blues' managed-care scheme in Michigan claims to have saved $2·57 million between April 1984 and September 1985 through pre-admission review of hospital stays, and between July 1983 and June 1984 saved $403,000 among enrollees at Ford and Chrysler through mandatory second surgical opinions.[2] North Dakota Blues saved $1·5 million after only five months of pre-admission review.[3] Experience elsewhere has been similar. The mayor of New York, Edward Koch, reported that the city had saved $1 million in 1985 by requiring municipal workers to get second opinions.[4]

---

[1] *Benefits Today*, 20 December 1985.   [2] *Ibid.*   [3] *Perspectives*, Fall 1985, p. 37.
[4] *Journal of Commerce*, 29 January 1986, p. 12A.   *Glossary, p. 113.

Integrating Supply and Insurance

On the supply side, the most significant response to pressure from purchasers and insurers has been the emergence of groups of providers who market themselves as cost-effective suppliers. Most have accomplished this by abandoning the traditional third-party payment role in favour of integrating health-care delivery with insurance. Vertical integration has taken three main forms: (a) HMOs; (b) PPOs; and (c) purchases of health insurance companies by hospital chains.

(a) Health Maintenance Organisations

The first HMO, the Ross-Loos Clinic, was founded in Los Angeles in 1929. Until the 1970s, the growth of HMOs was stifled by a hostile medical profession, but now there is at least one in every major metropolitan area and recent growth has been enormous. In 1972 there were 142 HMOs with 5·3 million members. Between June 1984 and June 1985 alone, membership increased by 21 per cent to 18·9 million and the number of HMOs rose by 28·9 per cent to 393 [Interstudy, 1985a].

There are four main types of HMO, the staff, group, network and independent practice association (IPA) models, though there are many hybrids. Under the staff model, doctors are usually salaried employees who provide care at a central location under the control of the HMO. Under the group model, the HMO contracts with an independent, often pre-existing, group practice at a single location. The physicians, both generalists and specialists, receive a capitation payment, usually paid monthly. The network model is like the group model except that the HMO contracts with more than one independent group practice. The IPA is an arrangement whereby the HMO contracts with a variety of doctors, most of whom are in solo practice, but some of whom may be in groups. They are usually paid by the HMO on a fee-for-service basis.

IPAs have been growing most rapidly, chiefly because they combine some of the advantages of traditional fee-for-service medicine with the cost restraint of other HMOs. In June 1985 they comprised 46 per cent of HMOs, with staff models 14 per cent, group 18 per cent and network 22 per cent. Traditionally, HMOs were non-profit but recently, largely in an effort to raise capital for expansion from the equity market, more have become for-profit. In June 1985, 36 per cent were for-profit, up from 18 per cent in 1981.

In the past, HMOs were typically local community health plans. Now there are 24 national firms with HMOs in more than one state, 10 of which opened for business between June 1984 and June 1985. The top seven HMO firms (Kaiser, CIGNA, Health America, Maxicare, US Health Care Systems, Prudential and United) account for over 80 per cent of total national HMO firm membership and 44 per cent of all HMO membership [Interstudy, 1985b].

HMOs depend for their success on being able to offer comprehensive services at a competitive price, by controlling utilisation, particularly of hospital stays. They use a range of strategies, including financial incentives to doctors not to over-use hospital facilities, informal peer pressure, formal utilisation review including pre-admission certification and concurrent review, lifestyle and 'wellness' education programmes for members, preventive health programmes, and searching out cost-effective providers.

Increased consumer power and lower costs

The economic significance of HMOs is that, because they threaten the position of established suppliers, they increase the bargaining power of the consumer and discipline the monopoly power of organised medicine. Goldberg and Greenberg, in a study for the FTC, found that the presence of an HMO reduced bed utilisation rates for members of Blue Cross as well as other organisations, produced an increase in the benefit levels of Blue Cross, and induced the Blues to found their own HMOs [1977b, pp. 110-18].

The HMO selects only those physicians who come up to scratch. Within the staff, group and network models, under which doctors are paid either a salary or a capitation fee, the financial incentive to over-hospitalise is removed. Under the IPA model doctors do have an incentive to over-use, but this is checked by utilisation review procedures. Often IPA doctors are also given financial incentives. Physician Care of Washington, DC, for instance, has a fixed-fee schedule of 85 per cent of usual, customary and reasonable (UCR) fees. Initially, 20 per cent of this nominal fee is withheld, and at the end of the year each doctor's utilisation record is examined. Doctors judged to have over-used services may receive only a proportion of the withheld sum. Unrepentent spendthrifts can be removed from the HMO panel.

Thus, the HMO enables the consumer to pay fixed monthly sums in return for comprehensive care from a set of known providers acting in an environment designed to promote cost-effective treatment. The HMO also eliminates the moral hazard faced by third-party insurers. It does so by eliminating the third party and acting as both provider and insurer.

The chief disadvantage of HMOs is that they have an incentive to *under*-provide medical services. A recent study of Seattle contrasts the health status of three groups of patients: (a) members of a local HMO; (b) fee-for-service patients required to share costs through co-payments or deductibles; and (c) fee-for-service patients with no cost-sharing. The study found that for most people HMO care saved money and may have contributed to better health. But low-income participants who began the experiment with health problems were in some ways in worse health than at the beginning. The authors of the study were uncertain about the reasons for this difference, but the HMO itself recognised that poor members were more likely to suffer from under-treatment and to remedy this weakness had introduced an 'outreach' programme of medical services for poor families [Ware *et al.*, 1986]. However, other studies have found no difference between the treatment of HMO and fee-for-service patients [e.g., Yelin *et al.*, 1985]. Several HMOs have erected internal safeguards against under-provision, but the subscriber's chief protection is his ability to take his money elsewhere. It is vital to maintain the consumer's freedom to choose, so that HMOs can flourish only by satisfying their customers.

(b) *Preferred Provider Organisations*

The recent rapid growth of PPOs has been largely a competitive reaction to the expansion of HMOs. As they lost customers, other suppliers came up with an alternative style of service which avoided some of the disadvantages of HMOs. The development of PPOs reveals how, once barriers to competition are removed, suppliers must re-direct their efforts into offering improved services to consumers.

An individual who joins an HMO pays a monthly premium and the HMO is at full risk for any health care required by the subscriber and included in the contract. The HMO 'locks-in' its subscribers, that is, if they go to a doctor outside the HMO panel they have no insurance cover. The PPO differs in two main respects.

First, the PPO itself bears no financial risk for the medical expenses incurred by subscribers. These are borne by the insurer, whether an insurance company or a self-insured employer. The providers are paid on a fee-for-service basis, at negotiated discounts, not by the individual patient, but by the insurer.

Second, the PPO does not lock-in subscribers. If consumers choose to use the services of a PPO doctor they are of course covered, but if they use an outside hospital or doctor they still enjoy cover, though possibly at a lower rate (perhaps 80 per cent or less). This is possible because PPOs have generally emerged as extensions of existing group insurance plans. They therefore represent an additional option available to subscribers. For the individual, the selection of a provider remains as it always was. He or she chooses a doctor or hospital and the insurer pays.

For the doctor or hospital the attraction of a PPO is the opportunity to increase market share. In addition, neither doctor nor hospital bears a financial risk. They are paid agreed discounted fees by directly billing the insurer, thus avoiding bad debts and the costly necessity to bill patients individually. Discounts range from 1 to 30 per cent of UCR fees for physicians, with an average of 20 per cent, and hospital discounts in December 1984 varied from 1 to 42 per cent.[1]

For the patient the advantages are that fees are reduced, and doctors usually conform to internal utilisation review which can protect the patient against poor-quality work. Above all, unlike the HMO subscriber, the PPO patient is not locked in to a particular set of providers, so the individual with a serious illness who decides to take no chances and opts to consult a specialist of national repute who is not in the PPO, can do so and still enjoy insurance cover.

For the insurer and purchaser (employer) the attraction of the PPO is that it is a halfway house between an HMO and traditional fee-for-service. It is a simple way for insurers or purchasers to identify cost-effective providers. It is also simpler to establish than an HMO, needing only an agreement about fee levels, utilisation review, and the details of claiming and direct billing. There is no capital expenditure. The PPO therefore provides a very loose, flexible formula, rather than a clearly definable organisational type. Indeed, it is not really an 'organisation' in the same sense as an HMO, but an agreement – a

---

[1] *Hospitals*, 16 December 1985.

contract – between providers and an insurer about fee discounts, utilisation review and methods of payment. For this reason the American Hospital Association insists on calling PPOs preferred provider *arrangements* (PPAs). They differ from the HMO also in not relying on total integration of the insurance and provider roles. The insurer continues to be a third party but the 'moral hazard' is reduced by the terms of the PPO contract. The beauty of the PPO is that hardly two are alike, so it is a formula which can be adapted to the widely differing circumstances of time and place.

Competitive promotion of PPOs

Because providers, purchasers (employers) and third parties (insurers and third-party administrators) all benefit from PPOs, each has had a hand in setting them up. Physician PPOs have usually been formed to maintain market share. Normally, a hospital builds the PPO around its existing medical staff (that is, all doctors with admitting privileges) and utilisation review machinery. Purchasers have usually started by identifying efficient doctors and hospitals and have then sought to incorporate them into their insurance plan by redesigning benefits to encourage subscribers to use the 'preferred providers'. The available evidence suggests that employers have been more interested in identifying physicians with a low utilisation record than those who are merely cheap [Lewin and Associates, 1984, III, 16].

Insurers and third-party administrators (TPAs) have also promoted PPOs. Indeed, the initial impetus appears to have come from TPAs like the Ad Mar Corporation in Santa Ana in California and Martin E. Segal and Co. in Denver [Lewin and Associates, 1984, III, 9]. In June 1985, TPAs had sponsored 12 PPOs. The Blues had founded 31 by June 1985, and are actively founding more. So too are the commercial insurers. By June 1985 they had sponsored 23 [AMCRA, 1985]. Employers are no less interested in PPOs. According to the survey of 861 companies carried out by A. S. Hansen, 12 per cent had PPOs in 1985, and 37 per cent of those without PPOs were considering them.[1]

There are no wholly reliable indications of the number of PPOs because they are still very much an emerging phenomenon. In 1975 there were none. In 1982 the AHA identified 33 PPOs in its first

---

[1] *Coalition Report*, February 1986, p. 7.

survey and by December 1984 it had found 115.[1] According to a survey carried out by the American Medical Care Review Association in June 1985, there were 334 PPOs, of which 229 were operational, with the remainder in the process of starting up. Membership figures are not available for all 229, but 75 PPOs were identified as having 3·4 million members [AMCRA, 1985]. According to the American Association of Preferred Provider Organisations, in November 1985 there were 325 in 36 states, with a membership of 5·5 million, up from 1·4 million in 1984.[2] From a survey of 98 PPOs, AMCRA found that they involved 176,000 physicians and 2,700 hospitals. A majority of PPOs were sponsored by physicians or hospitals (52 per cent of those reporting to AMCRA), with insurers (including the Blues and the commercials) supporting only 16 per cent of the total [AMCRA, 1985].

(c) *Hospitals as Insurers*

Both for-profit and non-profit hospitals have begun to move into insurance. The four largest for-profit hospital chains – Hospital Corporation of America (HCA), National Medical Enterprises (NME), Humana, and American Medical International (AMI), with a total of 100,000 beds in 744 acute-care hospitals – have each entered the insurance market in order more easily to continue gaining market share. They did not relish the prospect of trying to survive in a highly competitive market purely as hospital owners or managers. Humana offers Humana Care Plus, a conventional indemnity plan which has been available since January 1984. In August 1985 it had 315,000 subscribers in 5,000 employee groups. NME's HealthPace does not offer traditional indemnity insurance, but only HMOs and PPOs, while AMI's AMICARE relies wholly on PPOs. Launched in Miami in June 1985, through a health insurance company purchased in 1984, AMI hoped to have 150,000 subscribers within a year or so.

The two largest non-profit chains, Voluntary Hospitals of America (VHA) with 500 hospitals and American Health Care Systems (AHS) with 495 participating hospitals and 950 affiliates, are both entering the insurance field. VHA is offering PPOs through an arrangement

---

[1] *Hospitals*, 1 September 1985, pp. 68–73.

[2] *Hospitals*, 16 December 1985, p. 51; also *Health Care Competition Week*, 7 October 1985.

with the huge life insurance company, Aetna Life.[1] AHS has announced
the formation of American Healthcare Plans which will market HMOs,
PPOs and indemnity insurance [Kirchner, 1985, pp. 164–76].

Specialisation

Not only is insurance being integrated with provision, but segments
of the insurance role are also developing into specialised businesses.
The insurance function has been split into separate operations, with
new specialists emerging to compete with traditional insurers. Similarly, specialised suppliers, such as ambulatory surgery centres, emergency clinics, and home health agencies have emerged to compete with
hospitals.

(a) Insurers

Re-insurance companies have developed, specialising in stop-loss or
catastrophic coverage of the kind sought by employers under minimum premium plans. Sometimes a monthly limit is placed on the
company's total losses, and sometimes a limit per subscriber is calculated. This has led to the emergence of a new re-insurance institution,
the New York Insurance Exchange (similar to Lloyds of London)
[Etheridge, 1986, p. 7].

Third-party administrators (TPAs) have grown apace. In 1984 they
had 6,700 employer clients with a total of 5 million employees.
Specialised firms processing claims are also taking market share, offering the use of advanced electronic processing. Examples are the
National Electronic Information Corporation (NEIC) and IMX, which
is backed by a British subsidiary of ITT [Etheridge, 1986, p. 7]. They
can supply physicians with terminals in their office connected to an
on-line central billing bureau. Some specialise in the analysis of claims
records in the light of statistical profiles, others in claims validation,
and particularly double-checking whether bills match services
rendered. Hospital bills are notoriously inaccurate. In 1982 the Health
and Human Services inspector-general carried out a three-year study
of 34 Illinois hospitals and found that patients were 'often over-
charged'. In 1985 Equifax Services of Atlanta audited big hospital bills

---

[1] *Hospitals*, 16 December 1985, p. 42.

in all states at the request of employers and found that 97·2 per cent of the bills referred to them contained overcharging errors.[1]

Specialist data collection and analysis is also on offer. This can be of particular value to small employers with too few staff to make a viable insurance group. Specialist data analysts can arrange the pooling of several small firms to enable reliable premiums to be calculated. Peer review is now offered as an independent service by the utilisation review organisations (PROs) which have the Medicare franchises, as well as by other agencies [Etheridge, 1986, p. 7; Lewin and Associates, Chapter IV].

These new agencies have shaken up the industry and now the traditional insurance companies have had to set up specialist units to compete with the new TPAs, bill validation companies and data analysis organisations.

(b) *Providers*

Hospital inpatient care faces a challenge from ambulatory surgery centres offering one-day surgery. Their number has doubled since 1980 to 250 and it is estimated that there will be 600 by 1988. One survey of people who had received surgery in the two years up to 1985 found that 9 per cent had used a day surgery centre.[2] Hospital inpatient care is also under threat from home health agencies. Medicare-certified home health agencies grew by 17 per cent between October 1984 and 1985 to 5,825 agencies.[3]

Walk-in emergency clinics also offer competition with hospital outpatient departments and emergency rooms. They treat minor emergencies like fractures and carry out simple diagnostic tests. In 1985 there were 1,697, and patient visits were estimated to be up from 25 million in 1984 to around 44 million by the end of 1985.[4]

The for-profit hospital companies have been especially quick to respond to the reduced popularity of hospital inpatient care. The Hospital Corporation of America (HCA) increased its outpatient revenues in its US hospitals by 61 per cent in 1985, and is actively extending its role in the alternative services market. During 1985 it purchased three home care agencies [HCA, *Annual Report*, 1985]. AMI

---

[1] *Perspectives*, Fall 1985, p. 32.   [2] *Hospitals*, 16 December 1985, pp. 54–5.

[3] *Ibid.*, p. 52.   [4] *Ibid.*, p. 55.

is the market leader in day surgery centres, where over 750 medical procedures can be carried out at savings of between 30 and 50 per cent of hospital inpatient charges. It also has a fleet of mobile diagnostic vans, used by AMI facilities as well as others. This enables about 120 hospitals to share costly diagnostic devices such as CAT scanning units, cardiovascular ultrasound clinics and magnetic resonance imaging (MRI) units.

The Impact on Cost and Quality

The new climate of cost-containment has brought about a fall in hospital use. The number of hospital inpatient admissions fell by 6 per cent between 1984 and 1985, having fallen by 10 per cent from the 1981 peak figure. In both 1984 and 1985 the average length of patient stay fell by 4 per cent to around seven days. By the end of 1985 the national average 'hospital patient day-use rate' had fallen by about 18 per cent between 1983 and 1985 to around 950 patient days per 1,000 population. Hospital occupancy rates have also been falling. In 1981 hospital occupancy rates were 75·8 per cent; by 1985 the rate was 63·6 per cent.

This trend is in part the result of a shift to increased use of outpatient facilities. During 1985 the number of hospital outpatient visits increased by 7 per cent. Outpatient visits rose by 10 per cent from 220·9 million in 1981 to 243·4 million in 1985. Visits to doctors' surgeries also fell. Between 1983 and 1984 the average number of total patient visits per week fell from 125 patients per doctor to 119·4, a fall of 4·5 per cent [AMA, 1985, p. 3].

In 1985, hospital utilisation by Blue Cross and Blue Shield subscribers continued to fall faster than for the general population. In 1984 it fell by 7·4 per cent, and in the first six months of 1985 by a record 7·7 per cent. In the second quarter of 1985 subscribers were admitted as inpatients at the annual rate of 95 out of every 1,000 subscribers, compared with 103 a year earlier and 125 out of every 1,000 in 1975.[1]

According to the AMA, as a direct result of increasing competition, the real purchasing power of doctors' incomes fell during 1984. The average physcian's net income after expenses but before taxes increased by 2 per cent between 1983 and 1984, less than the rate of inflation [AMA, 1985, pp. 1,8-9].

---

[1] *Consumer Exchange*, January 1986.

Curtailment of expenditure naturally raises the question whether corners have been cut at the patient's expense. There are no systematic studies of the impact of the competitive environment on quality, though there are studies of the impact of diagnosis-related groups (DRGs) on the quality of Medicare. The hearings of the Senate Committee on Aging raised some doubts about the wisdom of rigid containment of medical fees [SSCA, 1985]. But this is a problem which has arisen because of the inflexibility of federal price-fixing by means of DRGs. In the private sector there is more flexibility. Moreover, insurers and purchasers are alert to these dangers and the emphasis has been placed on identifying cost-effective providers who cut costs without cutting corners. Utilisation review machinery is rapidly becoming more sophisticated in order to detect quality lapses. It is too early to draw conclusions, but so long as such monitoring continues there would appear to be no reason for alarm about the impact of competition on quality in the private sector.

IX. What About the Poor?

Gainers and Losers

We saw in Section VI how the cost of Medicare and Medicaid far outstripped expectations because payments were open-ended. As demand increased, Medicare and Medicaid simply had to pay. And, as we have seen, this has so far been overcome by pre-determining a fixed payment for each diagnostic group. Doctors now have to live within these cash limits. We also saw how hospitals initially reacted by shifting their costs onto other users, and how employers (who as the main purchasers bore the brunt of this cost-shifting) reacted. And as Section VIII showed, providers now face not only Medicare cash limits and a variety of Medicaid controls in some states, but also downward pressure on private sector prices due to competition. Again, the reaction of hospitals has been to try to shift their costs elsewhere.

The chief losers have been the uninsured. Private American hospitals have always treated a proportion of uninsured persons, either free of charge or at far less than cost. However, as competitive pressure has mounted, their willingness to do so has decreased, with the result that more uninsured patients have been sent to the county hospitals, which are funded from local taxes and function under an obligation to treat all patients.

This trend is a sharp reminder of the failure of the Great Society poverty programme. Before the mid-1960s there had always been considerable private charity care, but it was then felt that instead of relying on charity, people should be treated as of right. This has been accomplished for the elderly by Medicare, but the Medicaid scheme for the poor has failed to cover all who live below the federal poverty line. There is now a pressing need to devise new arrangements to enable low-income families and the unemployed to share in the purchasing power enjoyed by the vast majority of Americans as competition in health has re-emerged.

How Many Uninsured? – and Who Are They?

How many people in America are uninsured? The official National Health Care Expenditures Study of 1977 revealed that about 18·5

78

million people had been uninsured for a whole year, and an additional 16·1 million for part of the year. In any quarter, about 25 million people were uninsured [NHCES, 1985, p. 3]. This study may appear out of date but it is the most thorough investigation of the problem, and subsequent surveys suggest the numbers have not altered dramatically since then. The National Center for Health Services Research concluded in 1981 that there were about 27 million uninsured persons. The Washington-based Urban Institute put the figure at 33 million in 1982, and the Robert Wood Johnson Foundation found from its 1983 survey that 19 million reported themselves as uninsured [HIAA, 1985, p. 9].

Who are the uninsured? The likelihood of having no insurance for the whole or part of the year was well above the national average for the 19-24 age group, and for Hispanics, blacks and the poor [NHCES, 1985, p. 15]. About one-third of the uninsured are poor or near-poor; but half of the total are not, and have incomes at least double the poverty line [Wilensky, 1984, p. 54]. A major cause of the lack of insurance is unemployment. In a country where 85 per cent of privately insured people are insured through their employer, losing your job can mean losing your health cover. One study showed that about half the unemployed in Detroit had no health plan [Berki et al., 1985, pp. 847-54]. But not all employers provide health benefits, and of those uninsured persons in work, nine out of 10 were unable to obtain insurance through their employer. People working as servers in fast-food chains, for example, often have no health plan.

The chief difficulty is that Medicaid eligibility is strictly limited in many states. In 1982, 49 per cent of those with incomes below the federal poverty line had no public or private health insurance; 38 per cent were covered by Medicaid, and 13 per cent by employer health plans [Joe et al., 1985, p. 60]. But the uninsured are not left to go without health care altogether. 'Uncompensated care', which includes charity care and unpaid hospital bills, is provided on a large scale by the vast majority of hospitals. State and local governments supported public hospitals by grants worth about $9·5 billion in 1982, in addition to Medicaid. And private hospitals spent $3·2 billion on uncompensated care [Feder et al., p. 544]. Though occasional scandals occur, often leading to malpractice claims, people without insurance are not routinely denied emergency care. But it is common for patients who require expensive surgery to be transferred to the local county hospital where it will be provided out of public funds. Usually, patients are 'stabilised' at the first hospital they arrive at, and then transferred to the county hospital. The county hospitals, rather like the NHS, are a get-what-you-are-given system, with no choice of surgeon. Standards vary too. Some are very fine teaching hospitals but others are less proficient.

There is evidence that the 'dumping' of patients on county hospitals by private hospitals is growing and that standards of care in hard-pressed county hospitals may have suffered. In Chicago it appears that some patients have been transferred to the Cook County hospital before they were in a stable condition [Schiff *et al.*, 1986]. This raises urgent moral questions, but the main issue on which I focus is that of 'fairness'.

The Uninsured and 'Fairness'

The beneficiaries of uncompensated care are not a homogeneous group. Some are not poor, but have decided to remain uninsured or, if they have insurance, do not pay their deductibles or co-payments. But others live below the official poverty line and are therefore in need of help, while simultaneously the federal government subsidises higher-income groups through tax exemptions.

The cost in 1986 of federal tax subsidies to employer group health insurance has been estimated at about $49 billion [Enthoven, 1985a, p. 3]. In 1983, when the median household income was $20,885, a study by the Congressional Budget Office estimated that 88 per cent of tax-free employer contributions went to households with annual incomes over $20,000. The tax benefit averaged $622 per household in the $50,000–100,000 income bracket, and only $83 for those in the $10,000–15,000 range. This is both imprudent and unfair. It is imprudent because it encourages high-income groups to be careless about the cost of health insurance. According to Professor Enthoven, the message from the government to the well-paid is: 'Even if you buy wastefully expensive health cover, we will pay 40-50 per cent of the cost' [1985a, p. 6]. Open-ended subsidy is not only imprudent; it is also morally unjustifiable. If there is a case for subsidy, then it should go to people least able to buy health insurance.

These failings are widely acknowledged, but reform has not yet proved possible. There are a variety of proposals to cap the tax subsidy, including a 1985 bill sponsored by the Department of Health and Human Services and proposed in Congress by Senator Durenberger. It proposes to allow tax relief only on the first $100 of employer contributions for individual coverage, and $250 a month for family cover, index-linked to GNP. In addition, his proposed Health Equity and Fairness Act extends the tax deduction to individuals not in employer groups.

But the disadvantage of tax-cap schemes remains that people who cannot afford to pay health insurance premiums are left without subsidy. Professor Enthoven, among others, has therefore proposed that every person should be eligible either for a tax credit or a direct subsidy payable to qualified health plans. It would be worth 40 per cent of the premiums up to a limit of $60 per month for an individual, $120 for a couple, and $180 for a family at 1986 prices, again index-linked to GNP. According to Enthoven, this would have the effect of subsidising everyone, including those currently uninsured, and also making every beneficiary cost-conscious above the subsidy cap. At an estimated $47 billion in 1986, the cost would be a little less than the present subsidy [Enthoven, 1985a, p. 8].

Conclusion

The imposition by federal and state governments of price controls under Medicare and Medicaid, combined with downward pressure on private sector prices due to competition, has led to cost-shifting. The chief losers have been the uninsured poor. At the same time, the federal government subsidises employer group health insurance plans, which cover some of the best-paid people in the land. There is an urgent need to reform tax subsidies to give the unemployed and low-paid the power of choice that the present competitive market can make available to all.

PART 3

Lessons for Britain

X. The Challenge to the NHS

The Introduction singled out the three theoretical 'market failures' – professional monopoly power, consumer ignorance, and moral hazard. Having surveyed the American evidence, what should we conclude about recent orthodox 'market-failure' theory?

Professional Monopoly Power

The prevailing view of professional monopoly power rests on the claim that it is a *permanent* feature of health-care supply. According to Professor Culyer, for instance, it is a *universal* characteristic of all developed nations [1982, p. 37]. And Professor Maynard doubts whether liberals could ever secure the ending of the state-sponsored self-regulation which is the root of professional monopoly. The power of the doctors and the income losses they would suffer under competition, he says, 'make it likely that any market for health care will be dominated by monopolies' [Maynard, 1982, p. 508]. Writing in 1982, he feared that antitrust regulation to limit the doctors' monopoly in Britain would need to be 'substantial' and prove so difficult to execute as to be not worth attempting [1982, p. 495].

However, Section VII shows that the monopoly power of the American medical profession has been curbed by enforcing antitrust law through the Federal Trade Commission. Yet British supply-side theorists continue to assume that professional monopoly power will be a permanent feature of the future supply of health services. Indeed, Culyer has argued that professional monopoly power must be accepted as a fixed reality, and that consequently the state must be used as a countervailing force to limit the exactions of the organised profession and in particular to limit professional incomes [1982, p. 37]. Bosanquet advances a similar argument (above, p. 3). By such reasoning they infer that to limit professional salaries we must retain the NHS method of tax funding with provision in kind within a centrally-determined budget.

I have elsewhere questioned this theory in the light of historical evidence about the pre-NHS health market [1985b, Chapter 12]. Now it can be seen that countervailing-power theory is also contradicted by American evidence. Section VIII revealed that, once professional control of the supply of doctors was undermined, competitive pressures have curtailed professional power and produced widespread discounting of fees. Government price-fixing in the private sector has not proved necessary to contain professional incomes.

Consumer Ignorance

British market-failure theorists hold that one of the chief reasons for professional monopoly is the relative ignorance of the consumer. Advocates of competitive markets are scorned for assuming that the consumer can become sufficiently well-informed to select providers who will offer good quality service at 'reasonable' prices. Thus, because the consumer is too ignorant to exercise rational choice, competitive markets come to be dominated by producers. The 'marketeers' image', says Professor Culyer, 'of a prototypical consumer shopping around for the best quality care at the least price, and getting it, is not a phenomenon that is *anywhere* actually going to be observed' [1982, p. 39; my italics].

Before criticising this empirical generalisation about consumer ignorance, let me first make two general observations. Assertions about the relative ignorance of the consumer have a certain instant appeal because they rest on an apparently obvious truth. The very product being purchased from the doctor is information. At the diagnostic stage the patient reports symptoms in the hope that the doctor can explain them; and at the prescription stage the patient may want the doctor to set out the options. Similarly, at the active or therapeutic stage the patient will rely on the skill and experience of the doctor. Thus, to state that there is a knowledge imbalance is to state very little. Without it few people would take the trouble to see a doctor at all. The important question is whether the information asymmetry makes a competitive market impossible. And more relevant still to Britain: Is the information asymmetry so insurmountable a problem that it justifies the continuation of the monopolistic NHS?

A second common claim is that the consumer is not well informed about health *outcomes*. Ordinarily, a consumer can appraise the outcome of a purchase just as well as the supplier – does a bicycle work, a car drive well, a washing machine function as advertised? Health outcomes are said to be different. Neither 'before nor after the treatment', say Le Grand and Robinson, 'can consumers easily acquire information that will enable them to make an informed choice' [1984, p. 41]. There is an obvious grain of truth here, but much consumer uncertainty about health outcomes is a *general* uncertainty faced as much by the most skilled specialist as by the patient. When is it worth carrying out a coronary artery bypass operation? When should a tonsillectomy be performed? What is the most efficacious way to treat breast cancer? There is irreducible uncertainty about many such matters. Medicine is not an exact science. And to the extent that uncertainty confronts both parties, it is no reason for presuming the consumer to be especially ill-equipped to cope with choice. Moreover, it is no answer to uncertainty to put consumers wholly at the mercy of producers. The doctor may know relatively more than the consumer, but still faces too high a degree of uncertainty to be placed in an unassailable position. Yet, in reducing consumer choice, that is exactly what the NHS achieves.

Consumer Sovereignty in Practice

Moving on from general comments, I now summarise the evidence of how consumers have conducted themselves in practice. Does the evidence suggest that consumer sovereignty is unworkable? First, what happened in the past? My study of the British health-care market before the NHS shows that the deficiencies said to apply to all health-care markets were absent in this country. Working-class as well as wealthier consumers did 'shop around', making judgements about prices and the quality of service of particular doctors. They did not shop around as isolated individuals, but organised themselves in mutual aid associations – the friendly societies. Each branch elected one or more doctors and each had a disciplinary procedure which was used if doctors did not come up to the standard expected of them. Costs were contained and standards protected successfully [Green, 1985b].

The American evidence is similar. As we have seen, the assumption that consumer ignorance makes a competitive market impossible rests in large measure on a failure to ask *why* the consumer is ill-informed and especially to examine how much it is the result of professional restrictive practices. Since the FTC intervened to outlaw professional restrictions, American consumers have also been shopping around in well-informed groups seeking out the most cost-effective providers. Their groups are different from the mutual aid associations which flourished in Britain. In America, where over three-quarters of private health insurance premiums are paid by employers on behalf of their workers, the groups are typically organised around places of work. Employers often employ full-time specialist benefit managers to seek out the best price/quality bargains, and they have banded together in local health coalitions to seek out more systematically the cost-effective suppliers. Prudent purchasing is going on in America on a massive scale.

Can the competitive market in health care protect the consumer?

The consumer faces three main threats from any supplier of health services: overcharging, low-quality care, and unnecessary treatment or surgery. Has the competitive market proved capable of protecting people against these dangers?

Certainly the new competitive environment is already throwing up institutions which protect the consumer against overcharging. Doctors and hospitals are having to reduce prices to stay in business. There are also institutions which protect consumers against unnecessary surgery. Insurers insist on second opinions and pre-admission certification precisely to eliminate this menace. In addition, utilisation review machinery protects the patient against low-quality care. Concurrent review, which involves a nurse reviewer or physician adviser looking over the doctor's shoulder, protects patients against both unnecessary surgery and shoddy work. Insurers like doctors to get it right first time, because failure costs the insurer more. Utilisation review machinery generally is growing in sophistication and the efficacy of utilisation review methods is developing into one of the key factors taken into account by purchasers (employers) in choosing between this or that HMO, PPO or hospital. To retain or gain market share, providers have to do more than cut fees. They must show that their utilisation review machinery will not only control over-utilisation, but also detect the cutting of corners.

Competition has also made purchasers more selective in deciding which doctors to patronise. At present, market comparisons are based primarily on the cost and hospital utilisation record of particular suppliers. Quality comparisons are more difficult, but some comparative data are emerging. The Department of Health and Human Services has published the crude mortality rates of hospitals using data from Medicare peer review organisations [HHS, 1986]. But such material must be used with caution. Contrasting mortality rates during surgery with the frequency a particular procedure is carried out by an individual hospital has proved a more useful indicator of hospital performance. The less frequently a hospital carries out a procedure the more likely it is that patients will die on the operating table [Greenberg, 1984]. Such comparisons are in their infancy, but are gradually developing.

Developing 'brand loyalty' in health care

Another development is the emergence of 'brand-name' medical care. Sceptics will scoff that health care is not like soap. Nor is a Stradivarius! But the common feature is that 'brand' loyalty gives the producer an incentive to serve the consumer. So we see the emergence of large hospital chains, both non-profit and for-profit, as well as national HMO firms. All have much to gain by establishing a reputation for quality care at a competitive price. Those who recoil from this development should consider the alternative. If Kaiser, Humana or AMI were not free to try to build brand loyalty, we should soon see a return to the situation which existed before the recent re-awakening of competition in America, when there was only one 'brand' – the 'licensed medical practitioner'. The AMA's stubborn insistence on a single standard of training and competence was a monopoly strategy which denied choice and forced patients unwittingly into the arms of the less competent. So long as there is competition to give suppliers an incentive to improve, it is better to rely on non-profit Kaiser, or for-profit HCA, Humana or AMI, than to trust the 'professional' (for-profit) licensed-physician monopolist facing no such incentive.

These developments are now well under way, and we do not know exactly how things will turn out. The tragedy is that under the NHS we will never know or reap the potential for maximising the consumer's power to make well-informed choices. Only a competitive market can help us discover just how close to the ideal we can get. There is already enough evidence to refute the view that the health consumer is incapable of exercising rational judgement. Hence the folly of forcing people into the arms of an unwieldy, coercive, politicised, monopolistic NHS which brooks no alternative and blocks the emergence of innovations.

Moral Hazard

It is a commonplace that third-party funding creates a moral hazard, or a sense of financial irresponsibility. This charge applied to American health insurance until recently, as it still does to much private British health insurance, as well as to the NHS, where the absence of direct payment encourages demand regardless of cost. Some British economists have been impressed by this similarity and argue that the private and government sectors face the problem to a roughly equal extent. Thus, McLachlan and Maynard claim that:

'social institutions (the NHS and insurance companies, both private and social) reduce the price barriers to consumption and provide incentives for patients to over-consume (moral hazard) because a third party (the taxpayer or the insurance contributor) pays; and there are few incentives for decision-makers (doctors and managers of various sorts) to . . . ensure costs are minimised and benefit maximised' [McLachlan and Maynard, 1982, p. 554].

The key question is whether American evidence supports this view, and the answer is 'No'. The evidence which refutes the earlier claim of incurable consumer ignorance also refutes the claim that health insurance is unavoidably flawed by moral hazard. In America today, cost-containment is increasingly the norm.

But an important question remains. For many years health insurance in America did not promote cost-effectiveness. Why did insurers tolerate ever-rising costs for so long? In a competitive market this would normally offer opportunities for aggressive rivals to gain market share.

An important part of the explanation is the third-party status of the insurer. Until the mid-1970s the vast majority of Americans who had private insurance were covered through their employer's tax-subsidised health plan and most employers arranged comprehensive health benefits through an outside health insurance company. Looked at from the individual's point of view, there was not one third party but two. One was the employer, who in a competitive labour market did not want to upset his workers by scrimping and because of the open-ended tax subsidy was less conscious of health costs than other business expenses. The other was the insurer, who sold insurance cover to the employer. This divided responsibility created an especially strong moral hazard.

In addition, we know that the AMA applied sanctions to insurers who tried to contain costs and we know that this practice has persisted up to the present day. But we now also know that when the FTC intervened to outlaw the restrictions imposed on insurers by the AMA, the insurance industry began to compete, with the result that there are now a huge variety of cost-limiting developments on trial.

Moreover, the recent flowering of competition has directly diminished the problem of moral hazard. The growth of self-insurance (Section VII) represents an integration of the two third parties so that the insurer and the employer become one. Employers facing acute competition, such as American car manufacturers losing market share to the Japanese, could no longer ignore the cost of their health programmes and insisted that their insurance plans should include cost-containing elements. The insurance industry, supposedly flawed by irremediable 'market failure', found that it had to respond to market pressures and a wide array of cost-saving measures emerged.

The Public/Private Mix

So far I have argued that the failures said to characterise all health markets are not universal. I have also contested the theory that the NHS is an effective countervailing force to professional monopoly. There is another theory which is also susceptible to challenge.

It proceeds in three stages. It starts from the claim that the supply of health services is similar in both a market and NHS environment. It goes on to infer that changing the public/private mix will make no difference to health problems. And it concludes that all scholars must agree to focus their efforts on reforming the NHS. Some proponents even charge critics of the NHS with wasting scarce research time by continuing to study the potential of neglected competitive markets.

The most serious objection to this complacent approach is that it fails to confront fully the disadvantages of the NHS. Advocates of the theory are not blind to the defects of the NHS, but they do shrink from a properly balanced comparison with the market alternative. Indeed, two influential figures, McLachlan and Maynard, are so impressed by the *similarities* between the NHS and the market (as exemplified by the small British private sector and by American health care) as to claim that shifting the public/private mix 'does not remove regulation; it has a marginal effect and in reality merely changes its nature' [1982, p. 554]. This view is supposed to rest on the inherent properties of health care.

We now have enough hard evidence to dismiss such dogmatism by comparing the practical realities of imperfect markets with the realities of the imperfect NHS. In claiming that the best course for Britain is to concentrate on improving the NHS, McLachlan and Maynard turn their backs on a body of experience from which we have much to learn. By excluding the market option from consideration they assume that the NHS offers the best answer to at least three important questions:

1. What is the best way to allocate resources to health? Should funds be allocated according to 'need' or demand?

2. How do we ensure rapid adaptation to change so that our institutions match likely future requirements? Should we rely on 'planning' or leave room for 'trial and error'?

3. How best can the sectional self-interest of producers be prevented from damaging the general interest of consumers? Should we trust self-regulation with the state as monopsonist to prevent abuse, or rely on the promotion of competition?

'Need' or Demand

Some experts believe that future medical 'needs' can be predicted and the necessary hospitals, equipment and skilled staff can be calculated and duly provided. Without necessarily assuming this can be perfectly accomplished, adherents insist that allocation of resources by the state is preferable to market demand. The belief that medical 'need' can be measured rests on the mistaken view that *all* health care is like emergency care. But most illness is not life threatening. Equally important, there is no automatically 'correct' treatment which can be matched routinely with each patient's condition. Take a typical sequence of events. The patient experiences symptoms and goes to see a GP. The doctor may be able to diagnose the complaint immediately or require diagnostic tests to be carried out first. Then treatment may follow. There may be several courses of action available, each with its own advantages and disadvantages. There is time to think. Every such decision includes non-medical elements, such as cost (including time), the patient's preference for this or that degree or type of risk, and the patient's willingness to cope with this or that degree of pain or inconvenience.

Even a patient, told that he may have a year or so to live and that surgery may prolong his life by another year at the cost of great pain and disfigurement, may prefer to pay for home nursing in order to remain close to his or her family without putting an impossible burden of care on them. Consider breast cancer. A range of alternatives are available. The most radical is mastectomy, the surgical removal of the whole breast. The second is lumpectomy, or removal of the lump only, which is often preferred because it is less disfiguring. Other treatments include chemotherapy and radiotherapy, which produce unpleasant side-effects. Doctors dispute vigorously the relative merits of each alternative, and the evidence points to no objectively correct solution. A judgement has to be made about the treatment that best suits the patient and a vital part of this judgement can only be made by the patient herself. Coronary artery bypass operations raise similar questions, as do hip replacements and many other conditions. There is room for wide disagreement about the value and timing of such operations in any given case.

Faced with such choices, the consumer may choose to take no action at all because the proposed treatment entails unacceptable risks. Consider the case of Mrs Amy Sidaway, settled in February 1985 by the House of Lords. She had been experiencing persistent pain in her elbow and an operation was carried out to provide relief. It went wrong and she was left permanently paralysed on one side of her body. She attempted to sue the surgeon, arguing that if she had known the risk she would not have consented to the operation. The House of Lords came down on the side of the surgeon who contended that the risk of paralysis was one-in-a-hundred and that he was under no obligation to tell patients about risks as remote as that. The judges did not ask whether this contention would seem reasonable to an impartial observer, still less whether it would seem reasonable to the patient who bears the cost of failure, but asked instead whether other doctors conducted themselves in the same way. Because it was common for vital information to be denied as a matter of NHS routine, the Law Lords held that Mrs Sidaway had no redress.

But apart from the details of this particular case, a great many medical decisions are like the one that Mrs Sidaway would have faced if she had been fully informed by her surgeon. Knowing the risk of ending up in a still worse condition, some patients may decide to tolerate their pain, while others may choose to take a chance. Such judgements are plainly for patients to make, not for doctors, and any system which denies patients the right and responsibility to choose is deeply disrespectful of human life and dignity.

Cost of treatment: prices or arbitrary rationing?

It is also vitally important to recognise that the cost of treatment must be a factor in all medical decisions. There is a lingering feeling that sordid consideration of cost should have nothing to do with medical care. But the cost of care is always a factor which cannot be escaped, whether we like it or not. The only question is *who* decides. If patients do not choose, then the decisions will be made for them by the medical authorities or go by default. Under the NHS, such decisions are usually taken by doctors and administrators with the patient wholly or partially excluded. A striking example is access to kidney machines which is rationed by putting a 'use-value' on people's lives. If you are over 55 or have diabetes or a bad heart, or no dependants, or are not well known, it is likely that you will score a low 'use-value' and be allowed to die. Such rationing is an inevitable result of government decisions to allocate fixed annual sums for health care. In a market there is no such 'global' ceiling. If people wish to spend more by sacrificing other consumption they generally do so. And from year to year total expenditure can adjust to consumer preferences as insurance premiums rise or fall in response to demand and supply. The fatal flaw of the NHS is that it lacks any link between demand and budgetary allocation.

Nor are people denied treatment only because of budgetary constraint. The weighing of cost applies with special force to a growing range of non-invasive diagnostic tests. The view that 'anything which can be done should be done', which flows from seeing medical care as if it were all like emergency care, is not followed in reality. Judgements of utility are made by medical staff. For instance, if a person has persistent headaches for over a week, should a CAT scan be made? They are not only very expensive, but also clinically worthwhile in only a few cases. To the extent that cost explicitly determines whether to carry out the scan, the more power patients have over the decisions the more likely it is that their interests will be put first. It is true that the patient's decision may be distorted by insurance, just as it is distorted by the 'free' NHS. Generally, the bigger the out-of-pocket element in the insurance policy the more the patient will take cost into account, and *vice versa*. Such distortion cannot be wholly removed, but it is nonetheless preferable that the patient should have some say. The alternative is that other people will make the financial judgements, and almost certainly they will not have the patient's interests in mind at all.

No objective criteria for non-market allocation of resources

Some supporters of the NHS would agree with what I have just written but nonetheless insist that medical services should be allocated by the political and medical authorities. In doing so they put people at the mercy of decision-makers who cannot be expert in all the variables. Medical 'need' cannot be objectively measured or predicted, and resources allocated to match. Any decision about whether or not to proceed with some recommended course of treatment entails judgements which touch upon intimate personal matters such as willingness to endure pain, face risks and, not least, incur costs in the light of the alternatives on which the money might be spent. To the extent that non-medical judgements now form a vital part of all health decisions, there can be no experts. And to the extent that the NHS presumes medical decisions to be a matter of expertise, it is technically ill-adapted to cater for choice in a free society. Only a competitive market can reflect the increasingly complex character of medical decision-making.

Thus, the claim that resources should be allocated to health according to medical 'need' is in large measure misguided. But, even though the chief justification for government allocation of health resources is that medical 'need' should determine the NHS budget, in practice the sum assigned to health care is selected on grounds wholly unrelated to any calculations of medical 'need'. From the first days of the NHS in 1948, resources have been allocated to health according to criteria unrelated to either medical demand or medical 'need' – sometimes cut in an effort to control inflation, or perhaps raised when the economy was booming, or cut in order to spend more on defence or housing or social services.

Summary

The fixing of a total budget for the NHS by governments is undesirable for two reasons. First, factors wholly unrelated to either medical demand or 'need' have always been taken into account, and it is very likely that they always will. And secondly, insofar as the decision is based on measures of 'need' it will be ill-informed because medical 'need' is not objectively measurable. The general result in Britain has been that very much less has been spent on health care than would otherwise have been the case. And this is reflected in the evidence that, of all the industrialised nations, Britain is one of the lowest spenders on health as a proportion of GNP.

Why is market demand superior? It is preferable principally because the private judgement of each individual about how much to allocate to health is a better-informed judgement than any that can be made by government. In practice, a major part of each individual's decision will concern how much to spend on health insurance premiums, a decision usually taken once a year. Each person will have available to him a range of alternatives, such as several types of HMO, PPOs, and various indemnity insurance plans offering different degrees of comprehensiveness and varying levels of cost-sharing. The premiums will reflect the insurance companies' estimates of how much they will have to pay out in claims in the coming year and this will be based on what they paid the previous year. The consumer will decide how much he or she is willing to pay bearing in mind other demands on the household budget.

The total sum assigned to health by this multiplicity of private judgements more closely reflects what people wish to spend on health than any government decision ever could. General elections, for instance, do not allow a judgement to be made about the NHS alone, and even if there were a referendum on the single issue of the NHS, the decision being taken by the voter would be less well-informed than the annual selection a consumer makes between a range of insurance plans. But neither a general election nor a referendum can allow people to make sophisticated choices on behalf of their families about the type and extent of cost-sharing they prefer, or the degree of comprehensiveness they are willing to pay for, or the relative merits of HMOs, PPOs and traditional indemnity cover.

Innovation: Planning or Trial-and-Error?

Popular thinking about medical care takes it for granted that planning agencies will best devise the optimal institutions to supply health care. Again, it is not necessarily assumed that planning is without problems. But many British commentators believe that planning is superior to the market, which seems chaotic, with no uniform system and wide variations from place to place. Yet, if we analyse the improved institutional forms which have recently emerged in America, we must contemplate the possibility that freedom to innovate pays dividends foregone in the absence of a competitive market.

When the world is changing so rapidly, we should put as few obstacles as possible in the path of innovative individuals. It is not that governments are always wrong, but that the official faces different incentives from the free citizen. In a free society in which anyone can accumulate the capital to try out new schemes, the risk of personal loss helps eliminate less promising ideas. Government officials bear no cost for their failures and may therefore be less careful. Equally important, the scale of private experiments is limited, so that errors are less damaging and more easily corrected.

But the most serious objection to political or official resource allocation is that the raising of taxes to finance the NHS has had significant opportunity costs. If the money raised in taxes over the years had been left in private hands it would have been spent differently. It is by no means far-fetched to argue that but for the NHS Britain today would have more and better health-care services. Indeed, this conclusion is supported by a wealth of historical evidence which shows how promising British developments were stifled by the NHS and by contemporary evidence from America which suggests with still greater force that we have paid a high price for the National Health Service.

HMOs, for example, are widely respected, but could not have emerged under the NHS. When the first HMO developed in 1929, similar institutions had been in existence in Britain for some 50 years. They had been put under various disabilities by the 1911 National Insurance Act, and were finally snuffed out by the NHS in 1948 [Green, 1985a]. More recently, several new types of organisation have emerged in America. The growth of preferred provider organisations has been particularly dramatic, offering the advantages of HMOs without the restricted choice. One-day surgery centres and home health agencies have also developed to compete with hospital inpatient care. Outpatient departments are also under challenge from walk-in clinics offering emergency treatment and diagnostic testing. A wide range of experiments is being conducted by insurers to discover the best ways of promoting cost-effectiveness. Some involve cost-sharing of various types, whilst others prefer to rely more on control mechanisms which entail little or no cost-sharing. Gradually the best answers for differing circumstances are emerging by trial-and-error. Methods of identifying cost-effective suppliers are growing in sophistication, and new methods of improving the doctor's performance are being developed, such as concurrent review, second opinions and *profile analysis*,* by which the individual doctor's performance is contrasted with the median or the average. All these mechanisms add to the competitive pressure on providers to perform well. Purchasers are also struggling towards quality comparisons, though these are still at a very crude stage.

Faith in state planning presumes we can always foresee which institutions will prove valuable. But all the evidence suggests that we stand to gain as much from free experimentation in medical care as we do in other spheres of human endeavour. Our best hope lies with institutions as yet unimagined, and in remembering that some fruitful ideas seemed doomed to fail when first proposed.

Counteracting Self-Interest: Self-Regulation or Competition?

A final mistaken assumption made by supporters of the NHS is that it can control the abuses of self-interested producers better than institutions developed by the market. The interests of producers are always likely to clash with the interests of consumers. Contrary to the supposition that public servants will best serve the public, it is more realistic to assume that individuals employed in government retain their own interests, pursue them at work and give them priority over the interests of customers. The theorists of countervailing power may agree, but argue that the NHS controls the medical profession and thereby protects the consumer. I have suggested elsewhere [Green, 1985b] that it does so inadequately and at a high additional cost. The NHS has probably curtailed medical incomes, but it has not prevented doctors (especially GPs) from reducing their workload, or from elim-

---

*Glossary (under 'Utilisation Review'), pp. 114 and 115.

inating patients' rights of redress when mistakes are made. More important, the side-effect of NHS control has been worse than the original disease. The cost has been the arbitrary curtailment of medical expenditure within tight budget limits, and the patient has borne the brunt in poor services [Green, 1985b].

Summary

By displacing the market, the NHS has eliminated the competition which alone gives self-interested providers an incentive to serve their customers. Events described in Section VIII show that competition works in America to the benefit of the consumer. Prices are contained and doctors prevented from cutting costs by cutting corners at the patient's expense. American evidence also suggests that to encourage beneficial competition government must do more than merely stand back. It must intervene through antitrust law to ensure a competitive environment. I suggested in *Which Doctor?* how this might be accomplished in Britain, and here I will merely summarise the argument.

The orthodox medical profession has traditionally sought to differentiate itself from other practitioners of healing by imposing entry conditions on newcomers. Early on it sought a government seal of approval for its training requirements. Always justified as a way of protecting the consumer, professional entry restrictions can easily achieve the reverse, and the domination of the General Medical Council by orthodox medicine has had precisely this result. Widely-respected disciplines like osteopathy and chiropractic have been excluded, and the 'code of ethics' enforced by the GMC is in part a code of anti-competitive practices which reduces the consumer's ability to select from among alternative practitioners.

The risk of a patient falling into the hands of an incompetent practitioner justifies a government role in ensuring that certificates of qualification mean what they say, but it does not justify the imposition of a single national standard. For this reason I proposed the continuance of an official regulatory role, but not the present medical register which lists persons licensed to practise medicine. Instead of official licensing, a register should be maintained on which every person who wished to offer their services to patients should be required to record their name. They would be free to provide health care, but would be open to investigation by a new regulatory body which should replace the

GMC. Its powers would be limited to investigating and publicising. It would have no power to issue licences to individuals, nor to ban or withdraw official support from medical schools, nor to impose a universal code of ethics. Its role would be to expose those whose claims to expertise were bogus.

The medical profession's legal immunity from restrictive practices law under s. 13 of the 1976 Restrictive Trade Practices Act should be withdrawn. This would expose the profession and its anti-competitive restrictions to investigation by the Restrictive Practices Court, which presumes all such practices to be against the public interest unless the producer can show otherwise. The Office of Fair Trading is responsible for referring cases to the Court and should make a start with the General Medical Council's advertising ban, one of the chief barriers to competition.

Conclusion

The claim that the problems of supplying health care are the same in both market and NHS environments and that consequently the public/private mix makes no difference is untrue. Centralised budgets allocated according to 'need' ascertained by supposed experts – political, official or medical – fail to respect individual judgements about how much to spend on health, and have depressed health spending in Britain below the level free people would have chosen. Private demand is preferable to government-prescribed 'need'. Planning stifles innovation in medical services and, combined with the opportunity cost of a compulsory NHS and associated taxation, has forced Britons to put up with inferior health services.

Recent British history shows that the development of new institutions for the supply of primary health care in local health centres was stifled by the NHS [Green, 1985a]. And there is every reason to suppose that recent developments in American health care would have occurred here too, though with local variations.

Finally, competition protects the consumer more effectively than professional self-regulation, even if the state tries directly to contain medical incomes. Altering the public/private mix is very far from being irrelevant to solving our problems. Neither the NHS nor any market is free from imperfections, but markets have a self-correcting mechanism that helps to overcome problems which remain endemic within the monopolistic NHS.

XI. Conclusions and Recommendations

At the outset I asked whether Britain could improve upon the NHS, and in particular whether the promotion of competition between suppliers would benefit consumers. Both our own recent history and evidence from across the Atlantic show that competition improves health care. We have paid too high a price for the NHS, not only in the routine denial or delaying of treatment to hundreds of thousands of our citizens because of budget limitation, but also in lost opportunities for innovation because of centralised control.

My main purpose has been to survey the American evidence and to seek lessons for the reform of British health-care policy. The preparation of detailed proposals is a task for the near future, and I have room here for only a brief indication of the direction in which we should prepare to travel.

Beveridge's great hope was that the post-war welfare state would provide every person with security from want without destroying personal independence: 'in establishing a national minimum', he said, 'it should leave room and encouragement for voluntary action by each individual to provide more than that minimum for himself and his family' [Beveridge, 1942, p. 7]. We can now see that the welfare state in general, and the NHS in particular, has not achieved Beveridge's goals. Even the poor have not been fully protected, but – just as important – the NHS has failed to harness the natural desire of families to improve their lot.

The overriding aim of reform should be to achieve more nearly the twin aims of a national minimum and independent choice. This will require acceptance of at least three principles. *First*, the government should protect the poor, so that no-one is denied essential health care due to their inability to pay. *Second*, the government should not attempt to allocate resources to health care, because this will lead to a continuation of the pattern of underspending which has plagued the NHS since 1948, regardless of the political party in power. Instead, expenditure on health should as far as possible be a matter for the private judgement of each person or family, either in meeting out-of-pocket expenses or through insurance plans. *Third*, the government should promote competition between suppliers by ending the NHS monopoly. The NHS is already partially decentralised and in order to minimise short-run disruption there is no reason why the local district health authorities should not remain in existence, so long as they receive the bulk of their income only as a result of free choices by consumers from among an array of alternatives. In the early stages of transition from monopoly to competition, active government intervention to check the anti-competitive contrivances of the medical profession is likely to be required.

If these principles are accepted it should be possible to retain the chief virtue of the NHS, its aspiration of protecting the poor, whilst simultaneously enabling Britain to learn, not only from recent American experience, but also to absorb the lessons taught by our own history of providing medical care before the NHS began. The National Health Service as it stands, with its monopolistic obstruction of beneficial competition, its stifling of innovation, and its inbuilt tendency to under-provide for the sick due to budget constraint, is beyond redemption.

References/Bibliography

ABMS (1980): American Board of Medical Specialties, *Annual Report and Reference Handbook*, Evanston, Ill.: ABMS.

ACA (1986): American Chiropractic Association, *Chiropractic: State of the Art*, Arlington, Virginia: ACA.

ACNM (1982): American College of Nurse-Midwives, *Nurse-Midwifery in the United States: 1982*, Washington, DC: ACNM.

AHA (1977): *Advertising By Hospitals*, AHA Guidelines. Chicago: AHA.

AMA (1984a): *Medical Education in the United States 1983-1984, JAMA*, Vol. 252, pp. 1,513-1,601.

AMA (1984b): *Physician Characteristics and Distribution in the US*, Chicago: AMA.

AMA (1985): *Socioeconomic Characteristics of Medical Practice*, Chicago: AMA.

AMA (1986): *US Medical Licensure Statistics 1984 and Licensure Requirements 1985*, Chicago: AMA.

AMCRA (1985): American Medical Care and Review Association, *Directory of Preferred Provider Organisations and the Industry Report on PPO Development*.

ANA (1982): *Evidence to Sub-committee on Commerce, Transportation and Tourism of the Committee on Energy and Commerce*, House of Representatives.

Abel-Smith, B. (1976): *Value For Money in Health Services*, London: Heinemann.

Arnett, Ross H. III and Trapnell, G. (1984): 'Private health insurance: new measures of a complex and changing industry', *Health Care Financing Review*, Winter 1984, pp. 31-42.

103

Arrow, K. (1963): 'Uncertainty and the welfare economics of medical care', *American Economic Review*, Vol. 53, No. 5, pp. 941-73.

Avellone, J. C. and Moore, F. D. (1978): 'The Federal Trade Commission enters a new arena: health services', *New England Journal of Medicine*, 31 August 1978, pp. 478-83.

BHPr (1984): Bureau of Health Professions, *Report to the President and Congress on the Status of Health Personnel in the United States*, May 1984. US Department of Health and Human Services: No. HRS-P-OD 84-4 (2 vols.).

Bargmann, E. (1985): 'Washington, DC: the Zacchaeus Clinic – a model of health care for homeless persons', in Brickner *et al.* (eds.) (1985).

Berki, S. E. *et al.* (1985): 'Health insurance coverage of the unemployed', *Medical Care*, July, pp. 847-54.

Beveridge, W. (1942): *Social Insurance and Allied Services*, Cmd. 6404, London: HMSO.

Bosanquet, N. (1984): 'How to save the nation's health: the social market view', *Economic Affairs*, Vol. 4, No. 3, pp. 49-50.

Brickner, P. *et al.* (1985): *Health Care of Homeless People*, New York: Springer.

Brook, R. H. *et al.* (1983): 'Does free care improve adult health?', *New England Journal of Medicine*, 8 December 1983, pp. 1,426-34.

Buchanan, J. M. (1965): *The Inconsistencies of the National Health Service*, Occasional Paper 7, London: IEA.

Business Roundtable (1985): *Corporate Health Care Cost Management and Private Sector Initiatives*. (Results of the Business Roundtable Task Force on Health 1984 survey.)

CME (1964): Council on Medical Education of the AMA, *Medical Licensure Statistics for 1963*, *JAMA*, Vol. 188, pp. 877-901.

CME (1982): Council on Medical Education of the AMA, *Future Directions for Medical Education*, *JAMA*, Vol. 248, pp. 3,225-39.

Campion, F. D. (1984): *The AMA and US Health Policy Since 1940*, Chicago: Chicago Review Press.

Culyer, A. (1976): *Need and the National Health Service*, London: Martin Robertson.

Culyer, A. (1980): *The Political Economy of Social Policy*, Oxford: Martin Robertson.

Culyer, A. (1982): 'The NHS and the market: images and realities', in McLachlan and Maynard (eds.) (1982), pp. 23-55.

Culyer, A. and Posnett, J. (1985): 'Would you choose the welfare state?', *Economic Affairs*, Vol. 5, No. 2, pp. 40-42.

Dickerson, O. D. (1959): *Health Insurance*, Homewood, Ill.: Richard Irwin.

Enthoven, A. (1985a): 'Health Tax Policy Mismatch', unpublished paper, October 1985.

Enthoven, A. (1985b): *Reflections on the Management of the National Health Service*, London: Nuffield Provincial Hospitals Trust.

Etheridge, L. (1986): 'The world of insurance: what will the future bring?', *Business and Health*, January/February 1986, pp. 5-9.

FTC (1981a): *Statement of David A. Clanton, Acting Chairman FTC. Before the Senate Consumer Sub-Committee of the Committee on Commerce, Transportation and Tourism.*

FTC (1981b): *Physician Agreements to Control Medical Prepayment Plans*, 46 Federal Register 48982 (1981).

Feder, J., Hadley, J. and Mullner, R. (1984): 'Falling through the cracks: poverty, insurance coverage, and hospital care for the poor, 1980 and 1982', *Health and Society*, Vol. 62, No. 4, pp. 544-66.

Feldstein, M. S. (1967): *Economic Analysis for Health Service Efficiency*, Amsterdam: North Holland.

Ferrara, P., Goodman, J., Musgrave, G. and Rahn, R. (1985): *Solving the Problem of Medicare*, Dallas: National Center for Policy Analysis.

Frech, H. E. III (forthcoming): 'Monopoly in health insurance: the economics of Kartell *v.* Blue Shield of Massachusetts', in Frech (ed.) (forthcoming).

Frech, H. E. III (forthcoming): 'Preferred provider organisations and health care competition', in Frech (ed.) (forthcoming).

Frech, H. E. III (forthcoming): *Private and Public Health Insurance: Research and Policy*, Cambridge, Mass.: Ballinger.

Friedman, M. (1962): *Capitalism and Freedom*, Chicago: University of Chicago Press.

Fuchs, V. R. (1978): 'The supply of surgeons and the demand for operations', *Journal of Human Resources*, Vol. 13, Supplement, pp. 35-56.

Gabel, J. and Ermann, D. (1985): 'Preferred provider organisations: performance, problems and promise', *Health Affairs*, Vol. 4, No. 1, Spring, pp. 24-40.

Gensheimer, C. (1985): 'Reform of the individual income tax: effects on tax preferences for medical care', in Meyer (1985), pp. 53-66.

Gibson, R. and Reiss, J. B. (1983): 'Health care delivery and financing: competition, regulation and incentives', in Meyer (ed.) (1983).

Gibson, R. M., Levit, K., Lazenby, H. and Waldo, D. R. (1984): 'National health expenditures, 1983', *Health Care Financing Review*, Winter 1984, pp. 1-30.

Goldberg, L. G. and Greenberg, W. (1977a): 'The effect of physician-controlled health insurance', *Journal of Health Politics, Policy and Law*, Spring, pp. 48-78.

Goldberg, L. G. and Greenberg, W. (1977b): *The Health Maintenance Organisation and Its Effects on Competition.* (FTC Staff Report.)

Goodman, J. (1980): *The Regulation of Medical Care: Is the Price Too High?*, San Francisco: Cato Institute.

Goodman, J. and Musgrave, G. (1985): *The Changing Market for Health Insurance: Opting Out of the Cost-Plus System*, Dallas: National Center for Policy Analysis.

Green, D. G. (1985a): *Which Doctor?*, Research Monograph 40, London: IEA.

Green, D. G. (1985b): *Working Class Patients and the Medical Establishment*, London: Temple Smith/Gower.

Green, D. G. and Cromwell, L. G. (1984): *Mutual Aid or Welfare State: Australia's Friendly Societies*, Sydney: Allen & Unwin.

Greenberg, W. (ed.) (1978): *Competition in the Health Care Sector: Past, Present, and Future*. (Proceedings of a conference sponsored by the Bureau of Economics, Federal Trade Commission.)

Greenberg, W. (1984): 'Health care information in medical marketplace reform', *Society and Health*, December, pp. 21-3.

HCA (1985): Hospital Corporation of America, *Annual Report*.

HHS (1984): US Department of Health and Human Services, Division of Nursing, *National Sample Survey of Registered Nurses*, November 1984 (unpublished).

HHS (1986): *Statistical Outliers*. (A report of the Office of Medical Review, Health Standards and Quality Bureau, Health Care Financing Administration, HHS.)

HIAA (1985): *Source Book of Health Insurance Data 1984-1985*, Washington, DC: Health Insurance Association of America.

HRA (1982): Health Resources Administration, *The Impact of Foreign-Trained Doctors on the Supply of Physicians*, September 1982. US Department of Health and Human Services.

Harris, R. and Seldon, A. (1979): *Over-ruled on Welfare*, Hobart Paperback 13, London: IEA.

Havighurst, C. (1978): 'Professional restraints on innovation in health care financing', *Duke Law Journal*, No. 2, pp. 303-87.

Havighurst, C. (1982): *Deregulating the Health Care Industry*, Cambridge, Mass.: Ballinger.

Havighurst, C. (1983): 'The contributions of antitrust law to a pro-competitive health policy', in Meyer (ed.) (1983).

Havighurst, C. (1984): 'Doctors and hospitals: an antitrust perspective on traditional relationships', *Duke Law Journal*, No. 6, pp. 1,071-1,162.

Havighurst, C. (forthcoming): 'Explaining the questionable cost-containment record of commercial health insurers'.

Havighurst, C. and Kissam, P. (1979): 'The antitrust implications of relative value studies in medicine', *Journal of Health Politics, Policy and Law*, Vol. 3, No. 4, pp. 48-86.

Herzlinger, R. E. and Schwartz, J. (1985): 'How companies tackle health care costs: part I', *Harvard Business Review*, July-August 1985, pp. 69-81.

Hyde, D., Wolff, P., Gross, A. and Hoffman, E. L. (1954): 'The American Medical Association: power, purpose, and politics in organised medicine', *Yale Law Journal*, Vol. 63, No. 7, pp. 937-1,022.

Interstudy (1985a): *HMO Summary, June 1985*, Excelsior, Minnesota: Interstudy.

Interstudy (1985b): *National HMO Firms, 1985*, Excelsior, Minnesota: Interstudy.

Joe, T., Meltzer, J. and Yu, P. (1985): 'Arbitrary access to care: the case for reforming Medicaid eligibility', *Health Affairs*, Spring, pp. 59-74.

Joskow, P. (1981): 'Alternative regulatory mechanisms for controlling hospital costs', in Olson (1981), pp. 219-57.

Kessel, R. A. (1958): 'Price discrimination in medicine', *Journal of Law and Economics*, Vol. 1, pp. 20-53.

Kirchner, M. (1985): 'Will you have to join a hospital chain to survive?', *Medical Economics*, 25 November 1985, pp. 164-76.

LTV (1986): *Benefit Planning Kit*, Dallas: LTV.

Langsley, D. G. (ed.) (c. 1983): *Legal Aspects of Certification and Accreditation*, Evanston, Ill.: American Board of Medical Specialties.

Lees, D. S. (1965): *Health through Choice*, Hobart Paper 14, reprinted with a Postscript in Harris, R. (ed.), *Freedom or Free-for-All?*, London: IEA, pp. 21-94.

Lees, D. S. (1966): *Economic Consequences of the Professions*, Research Monograph 2, London: IEA.

Lees, D. S. (1976): 'Economics and non-economics of health services', *Three Banks Review*, No. 110, June, pp. 3-20.

Le Grand, J. and Robinson, R. (1984): *The Economics of Social Problems*, Second Edn., London: Macmillan.

Lewin, M. E. (1985): *The Health Policy Agenda*, Washington, DC: American Enterprise Institute.

Lewin and Associates (1984): *Synthesis of Private Sector Health Care Initiatives*. (A report prepared for the US Department of Health and Human Services.)

Maynard, A. (1982): 'The regulation of public and private health care markets', in McLachlan and Maynard (eds.) (1982), pp. 471-512.

McLachlan, G. and Maynard, A. (1982): 'The public/private mix in health care: the emerging lessons', in McLachlan and Maynard (1982), pp. 513-558.

McLachlan, G. and Maynard, A. (eds.) (1982): *The Public/Private Mix for Health*, London: Nuffield Provincial Hospitals Trust.

Meyer, J. (ed.) (1983): *Market Reforms in Health Care*, Washington: American Enterprise Institute.

Meyer, J. (1985): *Incentives vs. Controls in Health Policy*, Washington: American Enterprise Institute.

Meyer, J., Johnson, W. and Sullivan, S. (1983): *Passing the Health Care Buck*, Washington, DC: American Enterprise Institute.

NHCES (1985): National Health Care Expenditures Study, *Changes in Health Insurance Status: Full-Year and Part-Year Coverage*, Data Preview 21, Washington, DC: DHHS.

Newhouse, J. P. *et al.* (1982): *Some Interim Results from a Controlled Trial of Cost-Sharing in Health Insurance*, Santa Monica, Ca.: Rand Corporation.

Olson, M. (ed.) (1981): *A New Approach to the Economics of Health Care*, Washington: American Enterprise Institute.

Rayack, E. (1967): *Professional Power and American Medicine: The Economics of the American Medical Association*, Cleveland and New York: World Publishing Co.

Rosenberg, C. L. (1972): 'He challenged Aetna's hard-line fee policy and won', *Medical Economics*, 11 September, pp. 31–45.

Rottenberg, S. (1980): *Occupational Licensure and Regulation*, Washington, DC: American Enterprise Institute.

Rublee, D. A. (1986): 'Self-funded health benefit plans', *JAMA*, 14 February 1986, pp. 787–9.

SSCA (1985): Senate Special Committee on Aging, *Americans at Risk: the Case of the Medically Uninsured*, Staff Report and Hearing, 27 June 1985.

Schiff, R. L., Ansell, D. A., Schlosser, J. E., Idris, A. H., Morrison, A. and Whitman, S. (1986): 'Transfers to a public hospital', *New England Journal of Medicine*, 27 February 1986, pp. 552–57.

Seldon, A. (1968): *After the NHS*, Occasional Paper 21, London: IEA.

Seldon, A. (1977): *Charge*, London: Temple Smith.

Seldon, A. (1981): *Wither the Welfare State*, Occasional Paper 60, London: IEA.

Starr, P. (1982): *The Social Transformation of American Medicine*, New York: Basic Books.

Sugden, R. (1983): *Who Cares?*, Occasional Paper 67, London: IEA.

Sugden, R. (1985): 'Rejoinder', *Economic Affairs*, Vol. 5, No. 2, p. 42.

Sullivan, S. (1984): *Managing Health Care Costs*, Washington, DC: American Enterprise Institute.

USCC (1985): United States Chamber of Commerce, *Employee Benefits 1984*, Washington, DC: USCC.

Ware, J. E. *et al.* (1986): 'Comparison of health outcomes at a health maintenance organisation with those of fee-for-service care', *The Lancet*, 3 May 1986, pp. 1,017-22.

Weicher, J. (ed.): *Maintaining the Safety Net*, Washington, DC: American Enterprise Institute.

Wilensky, G. R. (1984): 'Solving uncompensated hospital care', *Health Affairs*, Winter, pp. 50-62.

Yelin, E. H. *et al.* (1985): 'A comparison of the treatment of rheumatoid arthritis in health maintenance organisations and fee-for-service practices', *New England Journal of Medicine*, 11 April 1985, pp. 962-67.

Zeckhauser, R. and Zook, C. (1981): 'Failures to control health costs: departures from first principles', in Olson (ed.) (1981).

Glossary

ADMINISTRATIVE SERVICES ONLY: An arrangement whereby an insurance company or other organisation pays claims and provides other administrative functions for a self-insured employer group.

CO-INSURANCE: A provision of insurance policies requiring the insured person to pay part of each medical bill, sometimes a fixed sum and sometimes a percentage of each claim, usually 20 per cent.

CO-PAYMENT: A type of co-insurance.

CONCURRENT REVIEW: A technique of utilisation review which involves a nurse reviewer or physician adviser in the employ of the insurance company double-checking the treatment recommended by doctors before and during hospitalisation.

DEDUCTIBLE: The (deductible) amount which must be paid by an insured person before insurance cover begins, like the 'excess' in British motor insurance. It is often an annual figure of about $200.

DIAGNOSIS RELATED GROUPS (DRGs): A method of classifying Medicare patients according to the condition responsible for their admission to hospital. The hospital is paid a fixed price for each of 467 DRGs.

INDEMNITY INSURANCE: An arrangement under which the insurer pays the actual expenses of the insured person for each claim, up to a previously agreed maximum.

MALPRACTICE INSURANCE: A type of insurance which covers doctors in the event of their being sued for damages by dissatisfied patients.

113

MINIMUM PREMIUM PLAN: An arrangement under which self-insured groups cover themselves against catastrophic losses, whilst remaining largely self-insured.

MEDICAID: A federal government grant programme in support of state schemes to provide medical care for the poor.

MEDICARE: The federal government scheme to provide medical care for the elderly.

MORAL HAZARD: The name given to the changes of attitude on the part of both doctor and patient which occur because the patient is insured. Once they have paid their premiums, patients may take the view that they want to 'get their money's worth' and consume more health care than they otherwise would; and the doctor, knowing that either a large company or the government is paying, may advise unnecessary treatment and inflate his bills.

NON-INDEMNITY INSURANCE (or SERVICE PLANS): Instead of paying a cash benefit the insurer undertakes to provide medical services in kind. The insurer pays the doctor direct or, in some cases, such as HMOs, the role of insurer and supplier are integrated.

PEER REVIEW: Utilisation review carried out by committees of doctors, and excluding outsiders.

PRE-ADMISSION CERTIFICATION: When the insurer gives permission in advance for treatment to be carried out.

PROFILE ANALYSIS: *see* UTILISATION REVIEW.

SELF-ADMINISTRATION: An arrangement under which a self-insured group provides all its own claims-handling services.

SELF-INSURANCE: An arrangement whereby a group, usually an employer, provides insurance cover from its own resources rather than by paying premiums to an outside insurer.

SERVICE PLANS: *see* NON-INDEMNITY INSURANCE.

UTILISATION REVIEW: The arrangements made to monitor the performance of individual doctors, including the intensity of their use of medical resources and the quality of care offered. It may occur before (pre-admission certification), during (concurrent review), or after treatment, as when the doctor's hospitalisation record is contrasted with some standard pattern or profile ('profile analysis'), like median-use rates.

Abbreviations

AAMC—American Association of Medical Colleges

AHA—American Hospital Association

AMA—American Medical Association

ASO—administrative services only

CON—certificate of need

CME—continuing medical education

DRG—diagnosis related group

FMG—foreign medical graduate

FTC—Federal Trade Commission

GME—graduate medical education

HMO—health maintenance organisation

JAMA—*Journal of the American Medical Association*

JCAH—Joint Commission on Accreditation of Hospitals

LCME—Liaison Committee on Medical Education

PPO—preferred provider organisation

PRO—peer review organisation

PSRO—professional standards review organisation

TPA—third-party administrator

UCR (fees)—usual, customary and reasonable (fees)